KETO S COOKER RECIPES

Delicious Low-Carb Ketogenic Diet Slow Cooking, 100 Weight Loss Recipes For Smart People

By Emma Green

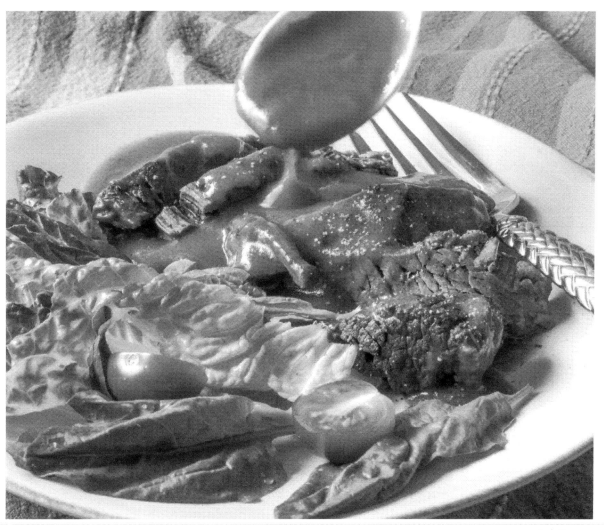

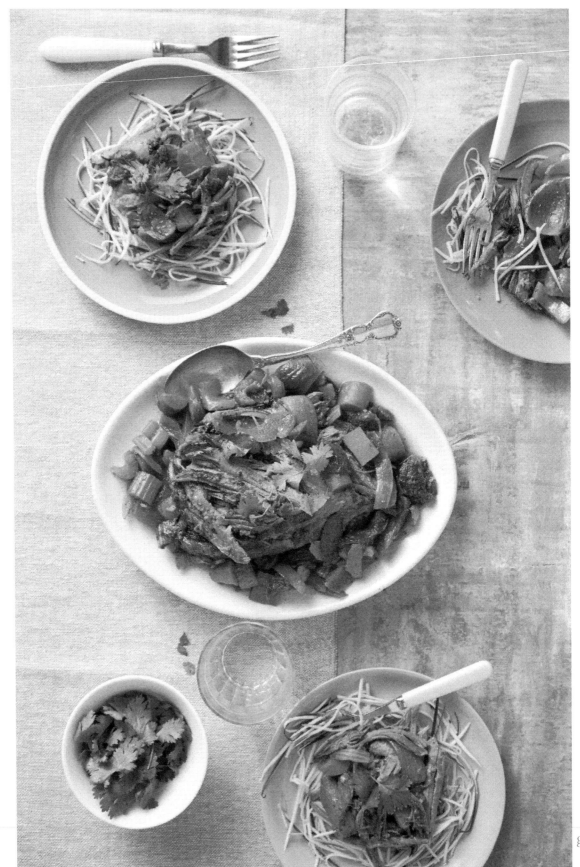

Table of Contents

Introduction

I want to thank you and congratulate you for purchasing the book, "KETO SLOW COOKIER RECIPES: Delicious Low-Carb Ketogenic Diet Slow Cooking, 100 Weight Loss Recipes For Smart People

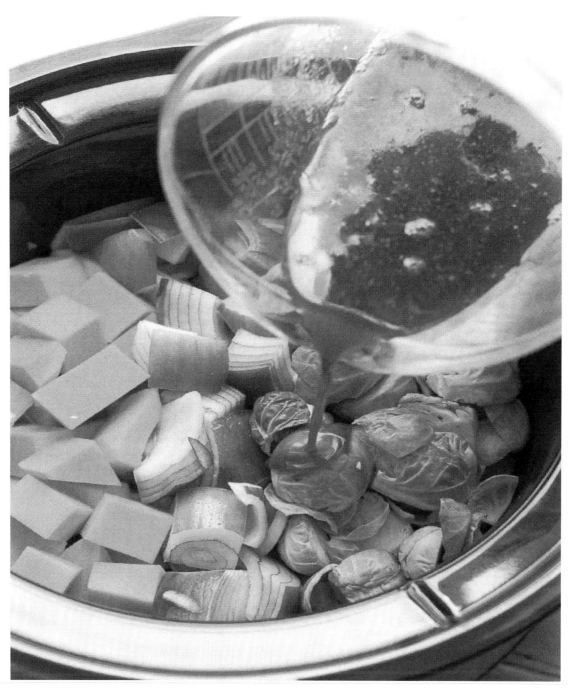

WHAT IS A KETOGENIC DIET?

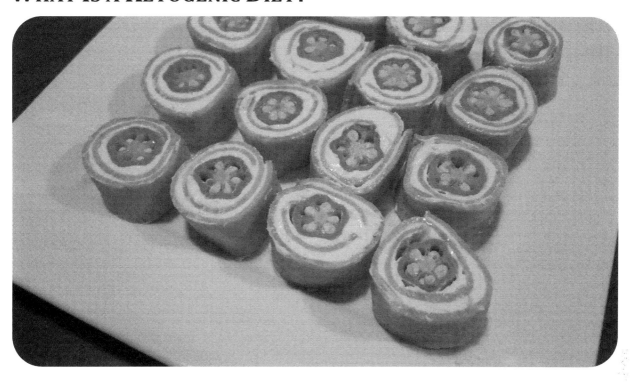

KETOGENIC DIET

Following the ketogenic diet allows you to change your body and adapt to a ketotic state of being. The ketogenic diet allows you to adopt a moderate protein, low carbohydrate and high fat content into your diet. Glucose is your body's main source of energy under normal circumstances, which is the broken down form of carbohydrates. Fats are then used as the body's main fuel source, which although sounds scary, is actually highly beneficial! If you're worried about your macros, don't be. A typical ketogenic inspired diet will consist of high amounts of animal fats as well as 20 -50 grams of carbs daily. You won't run short of proteins either, so that's no issue.

Though optimally, we'd want to cut back on carbs as much as possible, its presence in the ketogenic diet is only there to jump start the fat burning process and stabilize glucose levels in the body. Although you're cutting down on the amount of carbohydrates eaten, you aren't actually losing any calories. In fact, those are replaced by the high-fat content, which includes seeds, butter, nuts, avocados, cheese, eggs, fatty meats and coconut oil. Since they're fats, thy also play the role of increasing satiety. The levels of protein are also monitored so as to not get too high, otherwise it too can be converted to glucose – which makes carb cutting pointless.

THE BENEFITS OF KETOGENIC DIET

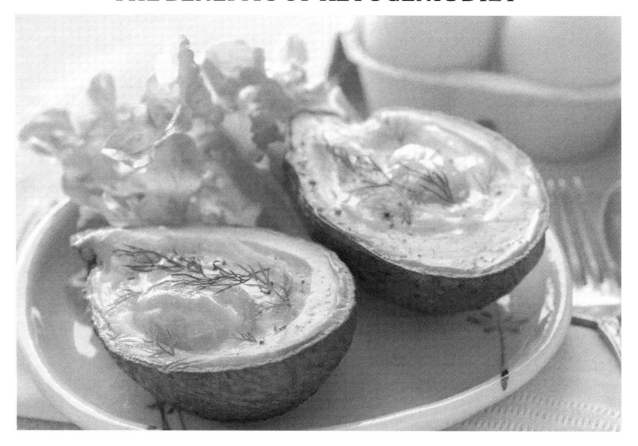

Once you've made the change from normal to keto, you'll start seeing a whole range of benefits associated with the switch. Your brain thrives on energy derived from ketones, and you won't have to worry about depriving it of anything. The benefits may include the following:

- A Decline in Risk Factors for Chronic Diseases
- Beautiful Skin
- Weight Loss
- Better Mental Clarity and Focus
- More Restful Sleep
- Staying younger
- Steady Energy

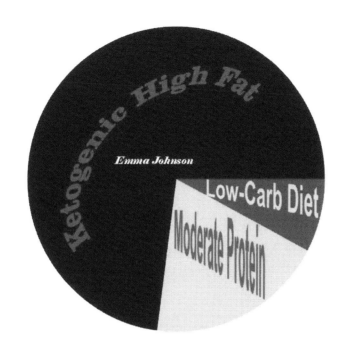

BENEFITS OF SLOW COOKER

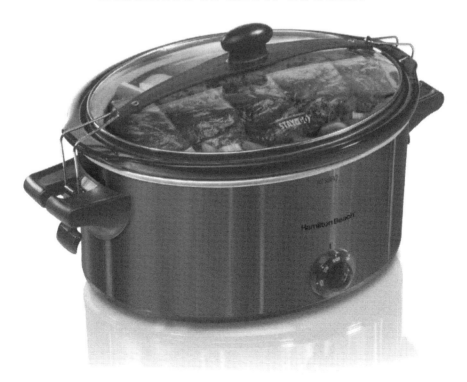

Spares your wallet: One way to save money is using a slow cooker, and that;s because they use so little energy. What's more, even cheaper veggies and cuts of meat taste even better when put into the slow cooker. Tougher meats —shanks, briskets, and chuck—break down very well into tender meals.

Better flavor: Long periods of cooking over slow heat and with the correct combination of spices are best for creating dishes that fill your mouth with flavour. Allow yourself to get the ultimate eating experience.

Time saving: Cooking from home is highl time consuming, but with the slow cooker, you only need to set it up and allow it to run itself. You could even prepare ingredients the night before and awaken to a lovely dish in the morning!

Convenient: Apart from saving time and money, the slow cooker is easy to carry with you, as it is often portable and handy. It also retains heat well, so no worries about icky microwaveables at your next dinner function.

Low heat: Especially on hot summer days, the slow cooker won't heat up your kitchen to unbearable scorching temperatures, so you can stay cool and classy!

Supports healthy lifestyle: High temperature cooking methods are damaging to your food's nutritional content, removing most of the antioxidants, vitamins and minerals while making an unhealthy amount of free radicals that precipitate disease. Low-heat is the best way to maintain this nutrition.

SLOW COOKER BREAKFAST RECIPES

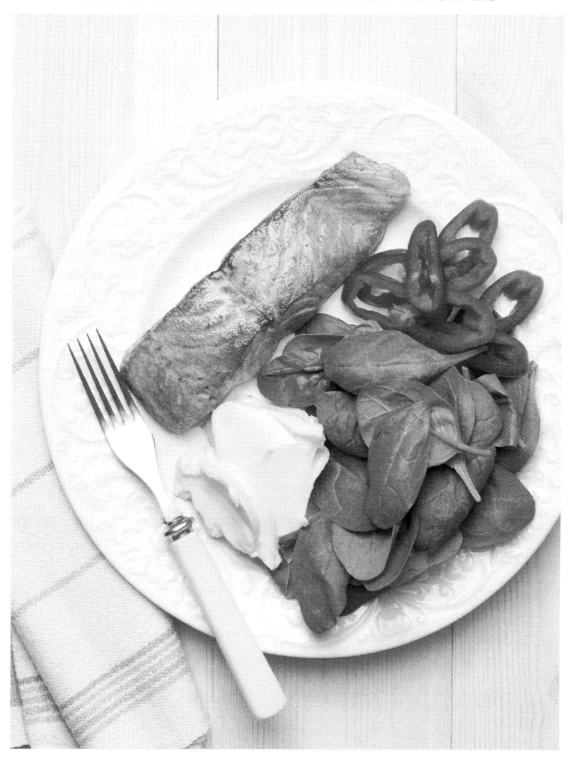

Parmesan Zucchini Paprika & Ricotta Frittata

Serve: 6

Time: 3 hours on high or Cook: 6 hours on low

Ingredients:

- 2 medium zucchini, shredded
- 1 teaspoon kosher salt, divided
- 1 tablespoon extra-virgin olive oil
- 12 large eggs
- 3 tablespoons heavy (whipping) cream
- 3 tablespoons finely chopped fresh parsley
- 1 tablespoon fresh thyme or 1 teaspoon dried thyme
- ½ teaspoon paprika
- ½ teaspoon freshly ground black pepper
- 6 ounces ricotta cheese
- 12 cherry tomatoes, halved
- ½ cup grated Parmesan cheese

Instructions:

1. In a colander set in the sink, toss the shredded zucchini with ½ teaspoon of salt. Let the zucchini sit for a few minutes, then squeeze out the excess liquid with your hands.

2. Generously coat the inside of the slow cooker insert with the olive oil.

3. In a large bowl, beat the eggs, then whisk in the heavy cream, parsley, thyme, paprika, pepper, and the remaining ½ teaspoon of salt.

4. Add the zucchini and stir to mix well. Transfer the mixture to the prepared insert.

5. Using a large spoon, dollop the ricotta cheese into the egg mixture, distributing it evenly.

6. Top with the tomatoes and sprinkle the Parmesan cheese over the top. Cover and cook for 6 hours on low or 3 hours on high. Serve hot, warm, or at room temperature.

7. Slice any leftover frittata into individual serving–size pieces and refrigerate in a covered container for up to 3 days.

Nutrition Value:

Calories: 291, Fat: 22g , Carbs: 4g , Protein: 18g

Cherry Tomatoes Thyme Asparagus Frittata

Serves 6

Time: 3 hours on high or 6 hours on low

Ingredients:

- 2 tablespoons unsalted butter, Ghee (here), or extra-virgin olive oil
- 12 large eggs
- ¼ cup heavy (whipping) cream
- 1 tablespoon minced fresh thyme or 1 teaspoon dried thyme
- ½ teaspoon kosher salt
- ¼ teaspoon freshly ground black pepper
- 1½ cups shredded sharp white Cheddar cheese, divided
- ½ cup grated Parmesan cheese
- 16 cherry tomatoes
- 16 asparagus spears

Instructions:

1. Generously coat the inside of the slow cooker insert with the butter.

2. In the slow cooker, beat the eggs, then whisk in the heavy cream, thyme, salt, and pepper.

3. Add ¾ cup of Cheddar cheese and the Parmesan cheese and stir to mix.

4. Sprinkle the remaining ¾ cup of Cheddar cheese over the top.

5. Scatter the cherry tomatoes over the frittata.

6. Arrange the asparagus spears decoratively over the top. Cover and cook for 6 hours on low or 3 hours on high. Serve hot, warm, or at room temperature.

7. Slice any leftover frittata into individual serving–size pieces and refrigerate in a covered container for up to 3 days.

Nutrition Value: Calories: 370; Fat: 29g; Carbs: 4g; Protein: 24g

Cheddar Spinach Breakfast Quiche

Serves: 6

Time: 2.5 hours

Ingredients

- 1/4 lb fresh spinach, chopped finely
- 1/4 tsp baking soda
- 1/2 cup almond flour
- 1 cup sour cream
- 8 eggs
- 1 1/2 cups cheddar cheese
- 1 large bell pepper, finely chopped
- 2 cups mushrooms

Directions

1. Butter or grease your slow cooker.

2. Stir the baking soda in with the almond flour.

3. Whisk the eggs together.

4. Add the sour cream, cheese, bell pepper, and mushroom.

5. Gently fold in the almond and baking powder mixture.

6. Pour everything into the slow cooker. Put the top on the crock pot and adjust the heat setting to high. Cook 2.5 hrs, remove and cut into 6 pieces. Serve hot and enjoy!

Nutritional Values

Calories: 268

Fat: 19.5g

Carb: 6.5g

Protein: 17.3g

Yummy Garlic Sausage & Egg Casserole

Serves: 8

Time: 4 hours

Ingredients

- 2 cloves garlic, minced
- 8 oz heavy whipping cream
- 1 head chopped broccoli
- 1/2 cup shredded cheddar
- 10 eggs
- 3/4 lb all-natural pork sausage
- Salt and pepper

Instructions:

1. Grease or butter the inside of your slow cooker.

2. Layer broccoli, then the sausage and finally the cheese onto the bottom of your slow cooker.

3. Whisk together the eggs, salt, whip cream, garlic, and pepper together separately.

4. Pour the mixture over the layered ingredients.

5. Cover your crock pot, adjust the heat to low and cook for four hrs.

6. Serve hot.

Nutrition Value

Calories: 377; Fat: 28.6g; Carb: 3g ;Protein: 25g

Shallot Parmesan Zucchini Asparagus Frittata

Serving: 6

Time: 1 hour 40 minutes

Ingredients:

- 12 eggs
- 1/4 cup fresh basil, chopped
- 1 cup parmesan cheese, grated
- 1 medium zucchini, sliced
- 8 oz asparagus, trimmed and cut into 2-inch pieces
- 2 medium shallots, chopped
- 3 tbsp olive oil
- Pepper
- Salt

Instructions:

1. Heat olive oil in a pan over medium-high heat.
2. Add zucchini, asparagus, and shallots into the pan and cook until asparagus is tender.
3. Remove pan from heat and set aside for 10 minutes to cool.
4. Spray slow cooker from inside using cooking spray.
5. Add cooked vegetables into the slow cooker.
6. In a bowl, whisk together eggs, basil, parmesan, pepper, and salt.
7. Pour egg mixture into the slow cooker over vegetables.
8. Cover slow cooker with lid and cook on high for 1 hour or until frittata is set.
9. Cut into pieces and serve immediately.

Nutritional Value : Calories 366 ;Fat 26.6 g ;Carb: 7.6 g ;Protein 28.6 g

Healthy Low Carb Walnut Zucchini Bread

Serving: 12

Time: 3 hours 10 minutes

Ingredients:

- 3 eggs
- 1/2 cup walnuts, chopped
- 2 cups zucchini, shredded
- 2 tsp vanilla
- 1/2 cup pyure all purpose sweetener
- 1/3 cup coconut oil, softened
- 1/2 Tsp baking soda
- 1 1/2 Tsp baking powder
- 2 tsp cinnamon
- 1/3 cup coconut flour
- 1 cup almond flour
- 1/2 Tsp salt

Instructions:

1. In a bowl, combine together almond flour, baking soda, baking powder, cinnamon, coconut flour, and salt. Set aside.
2. In another bowl, whisk together eggs, vanilla, sweetener, and oil.
3. Add dry mixture to the wet mixture and fold well.
4. Add walnut and zucchini and fold well.
5. Pour batter into the silicone bread pan.
6. Place bread pan into the slow cooker on the rack.
7. Cover slow cooker with lid and cook on high for 3 hours.
8. Cut bread loaf into the slices and serve.

Nutritional Value: Calories: 174 ; Fat: 15.4 g ;Carb: 5.8 g ;Protein: 5.3 g

Savory Creamy Breakfast Casserole

Serves 6 to 8

Time: 5 hours on low 3 hours on high

Ingredients:

- 1 tablespoon unsalted butter, Ghee (here), or extra-virgin olive oil
- 10 large eggs, beaten
- 1 cup heavy (whipping) cream
- 1½ cups shredded sharp Cheddar cheese, divided
- ½ cup grated Romano cheese
- ½ teaspoon kosher salt
- ¼ teaspoon freshly ground black pepper
- 8 ounces thick-cut ham, diced
- ¾ head broccoli, cut into small florets
- ½ onion, diced

Instructions:

1. Generously coat the inside of the slow cooker insert with the butter.

2. Directly in the insert, whisk together the eggs, heavy cream, ½ cup of Cheddar cheese, the Romano cheese, salt, and pepper.

3. Stir in the ham, broccoli, and onion.

4. Sprinkle the remaining 1 cup of Cheddar cheese over the top. Cover and cook for 6 hours on low or 3 hours on high. Serve hot.

Nutrition Value:

Calories: 465

Fat: 36g

Carbs: 7g

Protein: 28g

Delicious Bacon & Cheese Frittata

Serves: 8

Time: 2 hours 30 minutes

Ingredients

- 1/2 lb bacon
- 2 tablespoons butter
- 8 oz fresh spinach, packed down
- 10 eggs
- 1/2 cup heavy whipping cream
- 1/2 cup shredded cheese
- Salt and pepper

Instructions:

1. Butter or grease the inside of your slow-cooker.

2. Loosely chop the spinach.

3. Cut bacon into half inch pieces.

4. Beat the eggs with the spices, cream, cheese and chopped spinach. Then everything will be blended smoothly.

5. Line the bottom of the slow cooker with the bacon.

6. Pour the egg mixture over the bacon.

7. Cover the crock pot and adjust the temperature to high

8. Cook for 2 hours.

9. Serve hot.

Nutritional Value: Calories: 392; Fat: 34g; Carb: 4.5g ; Protein: 19g

Delight Breakfast Meatloaf

Serves: 8

Cook Time: 3 hours 10 minutes

Ingredients

- 2 lb ground pork
- 2 eggs
- 2 tbsp paprika
- 2 tbsp fresh sage
- 1 tbsp olive oil
- 1 diced onion
- 3 garlic cloves
- 1/4 cup of almond flour

Instructions:

1. Saute vegetables in the crockpot in the olive oil until brown.
2. Mix together the pork, eggs, sage, paprika and almond flour, thoroughly.
3. Add the cooked onions and garlic.
4. Shape the meat mixture into the shape of a loaf.
5. Put the loaf in the crockpot, cover with the lid and cook for three hours on low heat.
6. Serve in slices immediately, or save to serve at breakfast later.

Nutritional Value

Calories: 406

Fat: 28g

Carb: 5g

Protein: 32g

Low-Carb Hash Brown Breakfast Casserole

Serves 6

Time: 6 hours on low

Ingredients:

- 1 tablespoon unsalted butter, Ghee (here), or extra-virgin olive oil
- 12 large eggs
- ½ cup heavy (whipping) cream
- 1 teaspoon kosher salt, plus more for seasoning
- ½ teaspoon freshly ground black pepper, plus more for seasoning
- ½ teaspoon ground mustard
- 1 head cauliflower, shredded or minced
- 1 onion, diced
- 10 ounces cooked breakfast sausage links, sliced
- 2 cups shredded Cheddar cheese, divided

Instructions:

1. Generously coat the inside of the slow cooker insert with the butter.

2. In a large bowl, beat the eggs, then whisk in heavy cream, 1 teaspoon of salt, ½ teaspoon of pepper, and the ground mustard.

3. Spread about one-third of the cauliflower in an even layer in the bottom of the cooker.

4. Layer one-third of the onions over the cauliflower, then one-third of the sausage, and top with ½ cup of Cheddar cheese. Season with salt and pepper. Repeat twice more with the remaining ingredients. You should have ½ cup of Cheddar cheese left.

5. Pour the egg mixture evenly over the layered ingredients, then sprinkle the remaining ½ cup Cheddar cheese on top. Cover and cook for 6 hours on low. Serve hot.

Nutrition Value: Calories: 523; Fat: 40g;Carbs: 7g;Protein: 33g

Asparagus Crust-less Smoked Salmon

Serves 6

Time: 5 hours on low or 3 hours on high

Ingredients:

- 1 tablespoon extra-virgin olive oil
- 6 large eggs
- 1 cup heavy (whipping) cream
- 2 teaspoons chopped fresh dill, plus additional for garnish
- ½ teaspoon kosher salt
- ¼ teaspoon freshly ground black pepper
- 1½ cups shredded Havarti or Monterey Jack cheese
- 12 ounces asparagus, trimmed and sliced
- 6 ounces smoked salmon, flaked
- Generously coat the inside of the slow cooker insert with the olive oil.
- In a large bowl, beat the eggs, then whisk in the heavy cream, dill, salt, and pepper.
- Stir in the cheese and asparagus.

Instructions:

Gently fold in the salmon and then pour the mixture into the prepared insert. Cover and cook for 6 hours on low or 3 hours on high. Serve warm, garnished with additional fresh dill.

Nutrition Value:

Calories: 387

Fat: 33g

Carbs: 4g

Protein: 21g

Onion Broccoli Cream Cheese Quiche

Time: 2 hours 30 minutes   Serving: 8

Ingredients:

- 9 eggs
- 2 cups cheese, shredded and divided
- 8 oz cream cheese
- 1/4 Tsp onion powder
- 3 cups broccoli, cut into florets
- 1/4 Tsp pepper
- 3/4 Tsp salt

Instructions:

Add broccoli into the boiling water and cook for 3 minutes. Drain well and set aside to cool.

Add eggs, cream cheese, onion powder, pepper, and salt in mixing bowl and beat until well combined.

Spray slow cooker from inside using cooking spray.

Add cooked broccoli into the slow cooker then sprinkle half cup cheese.

Pour egg mixture over broccoli and cheese mixture.

Cover slow cooker and cook on high for 2 hours and 15 minutes.

Once it done then sprinkle remaining cheese and cover for 10 minutes or until cheese melted. Serve warm and enjoy.

Nutritional Value : Calories 296 ;Fat 24.3 g ;Carb 3.9 g ;Protein 16.4 g

Delicious Thyme Sausage Squash

Serves 4

Time: 6 hours on low

Ingredients:

- 2 tablespoons extra-virgin olive oil
- 14 ounces smoked chicken sausage, halved lengthwise and thinly sliced crosswise
- ¼ cup chicken broth
- 1 onion, halved and sliced
- ½ medium butternut squash, peeled, seeds and pulp removed, and diced
- 1 small green bell pepper, seeded and cut into 1-inch-wide strips
- ½ small red bell pepper, seeded and cut into 1-inch-wide strips
- ½ small yellow bell pepper, seeded and cut into 1-inch-wide strips
- 2 teaspoons snipped fresh thyme or ½ teaspoon dried thyme, crushed
- ½ teaspoon kosher salt
- ½ teaspoon freshly ground black pepper
- 1 cup shredded Swiss cheese

Instructions:

1. In the slow cooker, combine the olive oil, sausage, broth, onion, butternut squash, bell peppers, thyme, salt, and pepper. Toss to mix. Cover and cook for 6 hours on low.

2. Just before serving, sprinkle the Swiss cheese over the top, cover, and cook for about 3 minutes more to melt the cheese.

Make It Paleo Omit the cheese, and use a paleo-friendly sausage or diced ham.

Nutrition Value:

Calories: 502

Fat: 38g

Carbs: 12g

Protein: 27g

Tasty Greek Style Breakfast

Serves: 6

Time: 5 hours 20 minutes

Ingredients

- 8 oz spinach
- 3 cloves chopped garlic
- 12 eggs
- 1/2 cup milk
- 8 oz sliced crimini mushrooms
- 4 oz sun dried tomatoes
- 1 cup feta cheese
- Salt and pepper

Instructions:

1. Butter or grease the inside of your slow cooker.

2. Beat together the eggs, milk, garlic, salt, and pepper separately from the other ingredients.

3. Put in the sun-dried tomatoes, sliced mushrooms, and spinach, stirring well.

4. Put the egg mixture in the slow-cooker.

5. Top it off with the feta cheese. Cover the crockpot and set it on the low setting. Cook for five hours. Serve hot and enjoy!

Nutritional Value: Calories: 236 ;Fat: 15g; Carb: 7.3g ;Protein: 17.5g

Mexican Style Breakfast Casserole

Serves: 5

Time: 2.5 hours on Low, or 4.5 hours on high

Ingredients:

- 5 eggs
- 6 ounces pork sausage, cooked, drained
- ½ cup 1% milk
- ½ teaspoon garlic powder
- 2 jalapeños, deseeded, finely chopped
- ½ teaspoon ground cumin
- ½ teaspoon ground coriander
- 1 ½ cups chunky salsa
- 1 ½ cup pepper Jack cheese, shredded
- Salt to taste
- Pepper to taste
- ¼ cup fresh cilantro

Instructions:

1. Spray the inside of the cooking pot with cooking spray.
2. Whisk together in a bowl, eggs, salt, pepper, and milk.
3. Add garlic powder, cumin, coriander and sausage and mix well.
4. Pour the mixture into the slow cooker.
5. Close the lid. Set cooker on 'Low' option and timer for 4-5 hours or on 'High' option and timer for 2-3 hours.
6. Place toppings of your choice and serve.

Nutritional value: Calories: 320; Fat: 24.1 g; Carb: 5.2 g; Protein: 17.9 g

Almond Lemon Blueberry Muffins

Serves: 3

Time: 2-3 hours on High

Ingredients:

- 1 cup almond flour
- 1 large egg
- 3 drops Stevia
- ¼ cup fresh blueberries
- ¼ teaspoon lemon zest, grated
- ¼ teaspoon pure lemon extract
- ½ cup heavy whipping cream
- 2 tablespoons butter, melted
- ½ teaspoon baking powder

Instructions:

1. Add egg into a bowl. Whisk well
2. Add the rest of the ingredients into the bowl of egg. Whisk well.
3. Pour batter into lined or greased muffin molds. Pour up to ¾ of the cup.
4. Pour 6 ounces water into the slow cooker. Place an aluminum foil at the bottom of the cooker. Place the muffin molds inside the cooker.
5. Close the lid. Set cooker on 'High' option and timer for 2-3 hours.
6. Let it cool in the cooker for a while.
7. Remove from the cooker. Loosen the edges of the muffins. Invert on to a plate and serve.

Nutritional value:

Calories: 223; Fat: 21g; Carb: 5g; Protein: 6 g

Creamy Oregano Chorizo Mushroom

Serves: 8

Time: 4 hours 30 minutes

Ingredients

- 4 bell peppers
- 3 tbsp oregano
- 2 large onions
- 1 lb fresh mushrooms of any kind
- 1 lb cream cheese
- 1 cup milk
- 2 eggs
- 1 lb chorizo style Mexican sausage

Instructions:

1. Slice the bell peppers into thick slices.

2. Chop onion into large pieces.

3. Halve or quarter-chop mushrooms depending on preference.

4. Turn on slow cooker to high and begin to brown the chorizo, allowing the grease to bubble.

5. Cook onions, peppers and mushrooms for a few moments in chorizo grease.

6. Combine the creamed cheese, oregano, milk and eggs until blended smoothly. Pour milk and egg mixture on top of the meat in the crockpot and set to low heat. Cover and let cook for four hours. Serve hot and enjoy!

Nutritional Value: Calories: 516 ;Carb: 11g ;Fat: 42g;Protein: 22g

Healthy Veggie Omelet

Time: 1 hour 40 minutes

Serving: 4

Ingredients:

- 6 eggs
- 1 tsp parsley, dried
- 1 tsp garlic powder
- 1 bell pepper, diced
- 1/2 cup onion, sliced
- 1 cup spinach
- 1/2 cup almond milk, unsweetened
- 4 egg whites
- Pepper
- Salt

Instructions:

Spray slow cooker from inside using cooking spray.

In a large bowl, whisk together egg whites, eggs, parsley, garlic powder, almond milk, pepper, and salt.

Stir in bell peppers, spinach, and onion.

Pour egg mixture into the slow cooker.

Cover and cook on high for 90 minutes or until egg set.

Cut into the slices and serve.

Nutritional Value:

Calories: 200 Fat : 13.9 g ;Carb: 5.8 g ;Protein 13.4 g

Parmesan Sausage Mushroom Breakfast

Serving: 4

Time: On Low for 5 hours

Ingredients:

- 2 cups cooked ground sausage
- ½ cup chopped onion
- 1 Tbsp. parsley, dried
- 1 tsp garlic powder
- 1 tsp thyme
- 6 crumbled bacon slices, cooked and drained
- 2 cups organic chicken broth
- 1 cup red bell pepper, chopped
- ½ cup Parmesan cheese
- 1 cups heavy white cream
- 2 cups raw mushrooms, sliced
- Pepper
- Salt

Instructions:

Add all the above ingredients to a large slow cooker.

Cook on LOW mode for 4-6 hour. Make sure not to overcook or cook at too high heat or the cream will separate. Serve hot.

Nutrition Value:

Calories: 166

Fat: 15.5 g

Carb: 2.2 g

Protein 6.73 g

Arugula Cheese Herb Frittata

Time: 3 hours 10 minutes

Serving: 6

Ingredients:

- 8 eggs
- 3/4 cup goat cheese, crumbled
- 1/2 cup onion, sliced
- 1 1/2 cups red peppers, roasted and chopped
- 4 cups baby arugula
- 1 tsp oregano, dried
- 1/3 cup almond milk
- Pepper
- Salt

Instructions:

1. Spray slow cooker from inside using cooking spray.
2. In a mixing bowl, whisk together eggs, oregano, and almond milk.
3. Season with pepper and salt.
4. Arrange red peppers, onion, arugula, and cheese into the slow cooker.
5. Pour egg mixture into the slow cooker over the vegetables.
6. Cover and cook on low for 3 hours.
7. Serve hot and enjoy.

Nutritional Value:

Calories: 178 ; Fat: 12.8 g ;Carb: 6 g ;Protein: 11.4 g

Sausage & Egg Stuffed Mushrooms

Serves 6

Time: 6 hours on low

Ingredients:

- 1 tablespoon unsalted butter, Ghee (here), or extra-virgin olive oil
- 6 large eggs
- 1 pound mushrooms, stems minced, caps left whole
- 1 pound bulk breakfast sausage, or links with casings removed
- 1 cup chopped fresh kale
- 1½ cups shredded cheese of choice (see headnote), divided
- ½ onion, minced
- 2 garlic cloves, minced
- ⅓ cup chopped walnuts
- ½ teaspoon kosher salt
- ½ teaspoon freshly ground black pepper

Instructions:

1. Generously coat the inside of the slow cooker insert with the butter.

2. In a medium bowl, beat the eggs, then stir in the minced mushroom stems, sausage, kale, 1 cup of cheese, onion, garlic, walnuts, salt, and pepper.

3. Spoon the mixture into the mushroom caps and place each filled cap in the bottom of the slow cooker in a single layer.

4. Sprinkle the remaining ½ cup of cheese over the top. Cover the slow cooker and cook for 6 hours on low. Serve hot.

Nutrition Value:

Calories: 779; Fat: 61g;Carbs: 8g;Protein: 50g

Yummy Cauliflower Crust Breakfast Pizza

Serves 4

Time: 5 hours on low or 3 hours on high

Ingredients:

- 2 large eggs
- 3 cups riced cauliflower
- 1 cup grated Parmesan cheese
- 8 ounces goat cheese, divided
- ½ teaspoon kosher salt
- 1 tablespoon extra-virgin olive oil
- Grated zest of 1 lemon

Instructions:

1. In a large bowl, beat the eggs, then stir in the cauliflower, Parmesan cheese, 2 ounces of goat cheese, and the salt until well mixed.

2. Generously coat the inside of the slow cooker insert with the olive oil.

3. Press the cauliflower mixture in an even layer around the bottom of the cooker and extending slightly up the sides.

4. In a small bowl, stir together the remaining 6 ounces of goat cheese and the lemon zest. Dollop spoonfuls onto the cauliflower crust, distributing it evenly.

5. Put the lid on the slow cooker, but prop it slightly open with a chopstick or wooden spoon. Cook for 6 hours on low or 3 hours on high, until the edges are slightly browned.

6. When finished, turn off the cooker but let the pizza sit in it for 30 minutes before serving. Serve warm.

Nutrition Value:

Calories: 389;Fat: 29g;Carbs: 6g;Protein: 24g

Pecan Walnut Coconut Granola

Serves 10

Time: 2 hours on high

Ingredients:

- ⅓ cup coconut oil
- 1½ teaspoons pure vanilla extract or vanilla bean paste
- 1½ cups pumpkin seeds
- 1 cup unsweetened shredded coconut
- ½ cup almonds
- ½ cup walnuts
- ½ cup pecans
- ½ cup hazelnuts
- ½ cup sunflower seeds
- ½ cup erythritol or ½ teaspoon stevia powder
- 1 teaspoon ground cinnamon
- 1 teaspoon kosher salt

Instructions:

1. Set the slow cooker on high and let it preheat.

2. Put the coconut oil in the cooker. Once melted, stir in the vanilla.

3. Add the pumpkin seeds, coconut, almonds, walnuts, pecans, hazelnuts, and sunflower seeds. Stir to mix well, making sure all the ingredients are coated with coconut oil.

4. In a small bowl, stir together the erythritol, cinnamon, and salt. Sprinkle over the ingredients in the slow cooker. Cover and cook for 2 hours on high, stirring every 30 minutes.

5. Transfer the granola to a large, rimmed baking sheet and spread it out so it cools quickly. Serve immediately or store in a covered container at room temperature for up to 3 weeks.

Nutrition Value:

Calories: 495 ;Fat: 46g; Carbs: 12g; Protein: 18g

Low-Carb Cinnamon Almond Zucchini Bread

Serves 12
Time: 5 hours on low or 3 hours on high
Ingredients:

- ⅓ cup unsalted butter, melted and cooled slightly, plus more for coating the pan
- 1 cup almond flour
- ⅓ cup coconut flour
- 2 teaspoons ground cinnamon
- 1½ teaspoons baking powder
- ½ teaspoon baking soda
- ½ teaspoon fine sea salt
- ½ teaspoon xanthan gum (optional)
- 3 large eggs
- 1½ teaspoons pure vanilla extract
- 1 cup erythritol
- 1 teaspoon stevia powder
- 2 cups shredded zucchini
- ½ cup chopped walnuts or pecans

Instructions:

1. Generously coat a loaf pan with butter. (An 8-by-4-inch loaf pan fits nicely in my oval 6-quart slow cooker. Make sure your pan fits in the cooker before starting. No loaf pan? No problem. Use a round cake pan. Just fill it only about half to two-thirds full so the loaf has room to rise.)
2. In a medium bowl, stir together the almond flour, coconut flour, cinnamon, baking powder, baking soda, sea salt, and xanthan gum (if using).
3. In a large bowl, beat the eggs, then whisk in the melted butter, vanilla, erythritol, and stevia.Stir the dry ingredients into the egg mixture.Gently fold in the zucchini and walnuts.
4. Transfer the batter to the prepared loaf pan and spread it into an even layer with a rubber spatula or the back of a spoon.
5. Wad four pieces of aluminum foil into balls and put them on the bottom of the slow cooker insert. Place the filled loaf pan on top of the foil balls. (The foil balls should keep the pan raised about ½ inch from the bottom of the slow cooker so the pan doesn't get too hot.) Cover and cook for 6 hours on low or 3 hours on high.
6. Remove the pan from the slow cooker and invert the loaf onto a cooling rack. Let cool completely. Wrap in foil or plastic wrap and refrigerate. Slice and serve chilled.

Nutrition Value:
Calories: 213;
Fat: 20g;
Carbs: 5g;
Protein: 10g

KETO SLOW COOKER LUNCH RECIPES

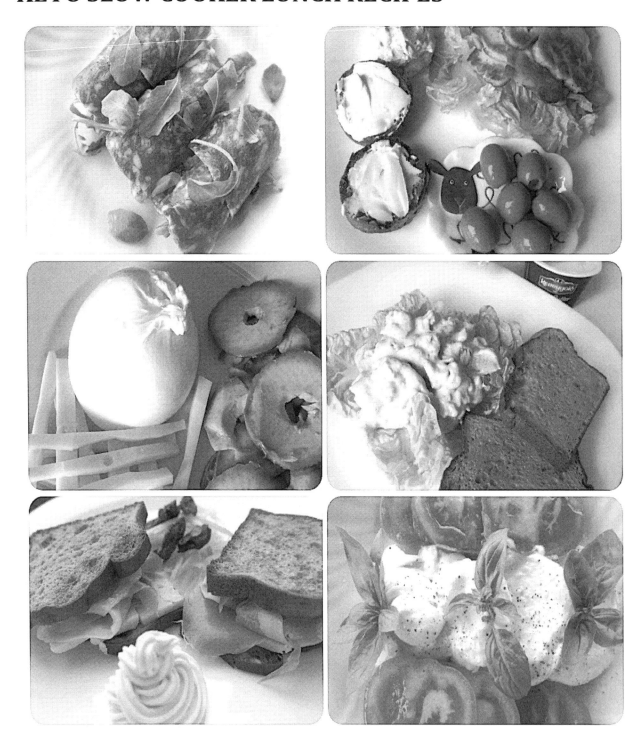

Butter Garlic Fish With Asparagus

Serves: 4

Time: 2 hours 20 minutes

Ingredients

- 4 haddock, cod or tilapia fillets
- 1 lb asparagus
- 2 tbsp chopped garlic
- 4 tbsp butter
- Spice as desired

Instructions

1. Cut out four pieces of aluminum foil, about twice the size of the halibut fillet.

2. Spice the fish, then divide them on their individual foil.

3. Place an even amount of veg with each fillet.

4. Top each fillet with a tablespoon of butter.

5. Wrap up each foil packet and seal the edges around the fish, vegetables, and spices inside to avoid letting out any of that flavor.

6. Place each packet in the slow crockpot, setting the heat to high.

7. Put the lid on, leave two hours.

8. Serve hot and enjoy!

Nutritional Value: Calories: 265 ; Fat: 12.5g ;Carb: 4.3g ;Protein: 33.3g

Yummy Cream Cheese Garlic Chicken

Serves 8

Time: 6 hours on low

Ingredients:

- 2 pounds boneless, skinless chicken thighs
- ½ cup (1 stick) unsalted butter, melted
- 12 ounces cremini or button mushrooms, halved or quartered
- 1 onion, diced
- 8 garlic cloves, minced
- 2 teaspoons paprika
- 2 teaspoons kosher salt
- 1 teaspoon freshly ground black pepper
- 1 cup chicken broth
- 8 ounces cream cheese
- 1 cup grated Parmesan cheese
- Fresh parsley, for garnish

Instructions:

1. Put the chicken pieces in the slow cooker. Pour the melted butter over the chicken. Add the mushrooms, onion, garlic, paprika, salt, and pepper and toss to coat the chicken with the butter. Cover and cook for 6 hours on low.

2. When finished, transfer the chicken and vegetables to a serving platter.

3. In a saucepan over medium heat, combine the chicken broth, cream cheese, and Parmesan cheese. Cook, stirring, until the cream cheese is melted and fully incorporated, about 5 minutes. Pour the sauce over the chicken and serve, garnished with parsley.

Nutrition Value: Calories: 495;Fat: 41g;Carbs: 6g;Protein: 26g

Delicious Italian Stuffed Meatloaf

Serves 8
Time: Cook: 5 hours on low or 3 hours on high
Ingredients:

- 1 pound (70% lean) ground beef
- 1 pound Italian sausage, casings removed
- 1 large egg, lightly beaten
- 1 cup sour cream
- ½ cup almond meal
- ½ onion, finely diced
- 4 garlic cloves, minced
- 2 tablespoons tomato paste
- 2 teaspoons dried oregano
- 1 teaspoon kosher salt
- 1 teaspoon freshly ground black pepper
- 1½ cups shredded fontina cheese
- ½ cup grated Parmesan cheese, divided
- ½ cup pitted, sliced olives
- Extra-virgin olive oil, for coating the aluminum foil

Instructions:

1. In a large bowl, mix the beef, sausage, egg, sour cream, almond meal, onion, garlic, tomato paste, oregano, salt, and pepper.
2. In a separate bowl, toss together the fontina cheese, ¼ cup of Parmesan cheese, and the olives. Lay out a piece of foil large enough to line the cooker and create a sling to help you remove the cooked meatloaf. Coat it with olive oil.
3. Form half of the meat mixture into a flat loaf in the center of the foil. Scatter the cheese and olive mixture in a strip down the center of the loaf. Top with the remaining meat mixture, enclosing the cheese and olives in the center of the meatloaf.
4. Sprinkle the remaining ¼ cup of Parmesan over the top. Using the foil sling, lift the loaf and lower it into the slow cooker. Cover and cook for 6 hours on low or 3 hours on high. Use the foil sling to carefully remove the loaf from the slow cooker and transfer it to a serving platter. Let the loaf rest for at least 5 minutes before slicing. Serve hot.

Nutrition Value:

Calories: 508
Fat: 40g
Carbs: 5g
Protein: 32g

Garlic Spice-Rubbed Pork Belly

Serves 6 to 8

Time: 8 hours on low

Ingredients:

- 2 tablespoons paprika
- 2 tablespoons onion powder
- 2 tablespoons garlic powder
- 1 tablespoon kosher salt
- 1 tablespoon freshly ground black pepper
- 2 pounds pork belly, thickly sliced
- 1 pound Brussels sprouts, halved
- 1 medium turnip, peeled and diced
- 4 bay leaves

Instructions:

1. In a small bowl, stir together the paprika, onion powder, garlic powder, salt, and pepper. Rub the mixture all over the pork belly slices.

2. In the bottom of the slow cooker, arrange the Brussels sprouts, turnip, and bay leaves in an even layer.

3. Lay the pork over the vegetables. Cover and cook for 8 hours on low.

4. Discard the bay leaves and serve hot.

Variation Tip Marinating the pork overnight in the spice rub means you have to plan ahead, but it makes for really flavorful meat. After completing step 1, wrap the pork belly tightly in plastic wrap, along with the bay leaves, and refrigerate overnight.

Nutrition Value: Calories: 848; Fat: 80g;Carbs: 14g;Protein: 18g

Mushroom Meatballs Ragout

Serves 4
Time: 7 hours on low
Ingredients:

- FOR THE MEATBALLS
- 1½ pounds sweet Italian sausage, casings removed
- 8 ounces ground pork
- 1 cup almond meal
- ½ cup pine nuts
- 2 cups finely grated Parmesan cheese, divided
- 1 large egg, beaten
- 1 teaspoon rubbed sage
- 1 teaspoon dried oregano
- ½ teaspoon kosher salt
- ¼ teaspoon freshly grated nutmeg
- TO MAKE THE MEATBALLS
- In a large bowl, thoroughly mix the sausage, ground pork, almond meal, and pine nuts.
- Add 1 cup of Parmesan cheese, egg, sage, oregano, salt, and nutmeg. Mix well. Form the mixture into 12 meatballs.
- FOR THE SAUCE
- ¼ cup (½ stick) unsalted butter, melted
- 1 (14.5-ounce) can diced tomatoes, with juice
- ¼ cup tomato paste
- ½ ounce dried porcini mushrooms, crumbled
- 1 teaspoon dried oregano
- 1 teaspoon dried thyme
- ½ teaspoon fennel seeds
- ½ teaspoon kosher salt
- ¼ teaspoon red pepper flakes
- 1 cup heavy (whipping) cream
- TO MAKE THE SAUCE

Instructions:

In the slow cooker, stir together the butter, tomatoes and their juice, tomato paste, mushrooms, oregano, thyme, fennel seeds, salt, and red pepper flakes. Nestle the meatballs in the sauce. Cover and cook for 8 hours on low. Just before serving, stir in the heavy cream. Serve hot, garnished with the remaining 1 cup of Parmesan cheese.

Nutrition Value:

Calories: 951; Fat: 70g; Carbs: 20g; Protein: 63g

Simple Healthy Meatballs

Serves: 8

Time: 5 hours 30 minutes

Ingredients

- 3 tbsp garlic salt
- 2 tbsp oregano
- 4 eggs
- 1 lb pork, hamburger style
- 1 lb beef, hamburger style
- 2 cups shredded parmesan cheese
- 1 can diced tomatoes (with the water)

Instructions:

1.   Turn the slow cooker on the low setting, then put the can of tomatoes with its water on the bottom.

2.   Mix the other ingredients thoroughly until everything is blended together well.

3.   Separate the meat into balls. They should each be around the size of a golf ball.

4.   Place the balls into the tomatoes at the bottom of the crock pot.

5.   Put the lid on the crock pot and adjust the heat setting to low.

6.   Cook for 5 hours .Serve hot and enjoy!

Nutritional Value: Calories: 429 ; Carb: 6g ;Fat: 32.8g;Protein: 41g

Tasty Jumbo Garlic Shrimp

Serves: 10

Time: 1.5 hours 20 minutes

Ingredients

- 4 oz butter
- 2 lb jumbo shrimp, peeled and deveined
- 8 tbsp olive oil
- 1 head chopped garlic
- 2 tbsp Creole seasoning
- Salt and pepper as desired

Instructions:

1. Melt the butter in the crockpot.
2. Combine the melted butter with the oil, garlic, and other spices.
3. Once everything is cooking nicely (about half an hour), add the shrimp.
4. Cover and set the slow-cooker to medium heat. Leave one hour.
5. Serve.

Nutritional Value:

Calories: 316

Carb: 3.3g

Fat: 23g

Protein: 22g

Chicken Soup

Serves 6

Time: 6 to 8 hours on low

Ingredients:

- 8 ounces boneless, skinless chicken thighs
- 3 cups chicken broth
- ¼ cup (½ stick) unsalted butter, cubed
- ½ small onion, diced
- 2 garlic cloves, minced
- 1 teaspoon kosher salt
- ½ teaspoon freshly ground black pepper
- 1¼ cups heavy (whipping) cream

Instructions:

1. In the slow cooker, combine the chicken, chicken broth, butter, onion, garlic, salt, and pepper. Cover and cook for 6 to 8 hours on low.

2. Remove the chicken from the soup and chop or shred it. Stir the chicken back into the soup, along with the heavy cream. Serve hot.

Nutrition Value:

Calories: 373

Fat: 33g

Carbs: 7g

Protein: 14g

Garlic Celery Spicy Beef

Serves 8

Time: 8 hours on low

Ingredients:

- 2½ pounds (70% lean) ground beef
- 2 teaspoons kosher salt
- 1 teaspoon freshly ground black pepper
- 1 red onion, diced, divided
- 6 garlic cloves, minced
- 3 celery stalks, diced
- ¼ cup sliced jalapeño peppers
- 1 (7-ounce) can diced fire-roasted green chiles, drained
- 1 (28-ounce) can diced tomatoes, with juice
- 1 (6-ounce) can tomato paste
- 3 tablespoons chili powder
- 3 tablespoons ground cumin
- 1 teaspoon dried oregano
- 1 bay leaf

Instructions:

Shredded Cheddar cheese, for garnish

Sour cream, for garnish

Sliced avocado, for garnish

1. Heat a large skillet over medium-high heat. Add the beef, salt, and pepper and sauté until the beef is browned, about 5 minutes. Transfer to the slow cooker.

2. Stir in the onion, garlic, celery, jalapeños, green chiles, tomatoes and their juice, tomato paste, chili powder, cumin, oregano, and bay leaf. Cover and cook for 8 hours on low.

3. Discard the bay leaf and serve hot, garnished with Cheddar cheese, sour cream, and avocado.

Nutrition Value:

Calories: 685; Fat: 58g;Carbs: 15g;Protein: 28g

Basil Ground Turkey Meatballs in Sauce

Serves 8
Time: 7 hours on low
Ingredients:

- FOR THE SAUCE
- ¼ cup (½ stick) unsalted butter, melted
- 1 (14.5-ounce) can crushed tomatoes
- 1 tablespoon extra-virgin olive oil
- 2 garlic cloves, minced
- 2 teaspoons dried basil
- 1 teaspoon dried parsley
- 1 teaspoon kosher salt
- ½ teaspoon freshly ground black pepper
- 1 cup heavy (whipping) cream
- TO MAKE THE SAUCE
- In the slow cooker, stir together the butter, tomatoes, olive oil, garlic, basil, parsley, salt, and pepper.
- FOR THE MEATBALLS
- 2 large eggs
- 2 cups riced cauliflower
- ½ cup almond meal
- 2 cups grated Parmesan cheese, divided
- 2 tablespoons Italian seasoning
- 1 teaspoon kosher salt
- ½ teaspoon freshly ground black pepper
- ½ teaspoon garlic powder
- 12 ounces ground turkey
- 1 pound Italian sausage, casings removed
- 8 ounces fontina cheese, cut into 24 cubes

TO MAKE THE MEATBALLS

Instructions:

1. In a large bowl, beat the eggs, then whisk in the cauliflower rice, almond meal, 1 cup of Parmesan cheese, Italian seasoning, salt, pepper, and garlic powder.
2. Add the turkey and sausage and mix to combine. Form the mixture into 24 (1-inch) balls.
3. Stuff a cheese cube into the center of each meatball and press the meat mixture around it so it is fully encased. Place the stuffed meatballs in the slow cooker. Cover and cook for 7 hours on low.
4. Just before serving, stir the heavy cream into the sauce. Serve hot, garnished with the remaining 1 cup of Parmesan cheese.

Nutrition Value:
Calories: 633, Fat: 50g, Carbs: 9g, Protein: 39g

Garlic Onion Lemongrass Pork

Serves 6

Time: 8 hours on low

Ingredients:

- ¼ cup coconut oil, melted
- 1 tablespoon apple cider vinegar
- 3 tablespoons minced lemongrass (white part only)
- 3 garlic cloves, minced
- 2 teaspoons kosher salt
- 1 teaspoon freshly ground black pepper
- 2 pounds boneless pork shoulder or butt roast, top fatty layer scored in a crisscross pattern
- 1 onion, sliced
- 1 (2-inch) piece fresh ginger, peeled and cut into thin slices
- 1 (14-ounce) can coconut milk

Instructions:

1. In a small bowl, stir together the coconut oil, cider vinegar, lemongrass, garlic, salt, and pepper.

2. Place the pork in a baking dish and rub the seasoning mixture all over it. Cover and refrigerate overnight.

3. In the morning, remove the pork from the refrigerator 30 to 60 minutes before you plan to cook it so it can come to room temperature. You could also complete the next step and then set a delay timer to start the slow cooker 30 to 60 minutes later, if you prefer.

4. Cover the bottom of the slow cooker with the onion and ginger slices in an even layer. Top with the marinated pork, along with any accumulated juices in the dish. Pour the coconut milk over the top. Cover and cook for 8 hours on low.

5. Shred the meat using two forks. Serve immediately, refrigerate for up to 3 days, or freeze for up to 3 months.

Nutrition Value: Calories: 547;Fat: 43g;Carbs: 6g;Protein: 34g

Leek Bacon Chicken Chowder

Serves 6

Time: 8 hours on low

Ingredients:

- 12 ounces bacon
- 4 tablespoons (½ stick) unsalted butter or Ghee (here), at room temperature, divided
- 12 ounces boneless, skinless chicken breast, diced
- 6 ounces cremini mushrooms, sliced
- 2 celery stalks, diced
- 1 leek (white and pale green parts), halved lengthwise and thinly sliced crosswise
- 1 onion, thinly sliced
- 1 shallot, finely chopped
- 4 garlic cloves, minced
- 1 tablespoon minced fresh thyme
- 1 teaspoon kosher salt
- 1 teaspoon freshly ground black pepper
- 2 cups chicken broth
- 1 cup heavy (whipping) cream
- 8 ounces cream cheese, at room temperature

Instructions:

1. In a large skillet, cook the bacon over medium heat until crisp. Transfer to a paper towel–lined plate to drain. Crumble into small pieces and set aside.

2. Spread 2 tablespoons of butter over the bottom of the slow cooker insert.

3. Add the chicken, cooked bacon, mushrooms, celery, leek, onion, shallot, garlic, thyme, salt, and pepper.

4. In a medium bowl, whisk together the chicken broth, heavy cream, cream cheese, and remaining 2 tablespoons of butter until well combined and smooth. Pour the mixture over the ingredients in the slow cooker and stir to mix. Cover and cook for 8 hours on low. Serve hot.

Nutrition Value: Calories: 573;Fat: 45g;Carbs: 12g; Protein: 31g

Low-carb Lamb Stew

Serves: 4

Time: 6 hours 20 minutes

Ingredients:

- 1 lb all-natural Lamb, chunked for stew
- One short can (6 oz) tomato paste
- 1 large chopped onion
- 3 garlic cloves
- 3 cups green beans
- 3 tbsp thyme
- 2 bay leaves
- 3 diced celery stalks

Instructions:

1.   Put all ingredients into the slow-cooker and mix well.

2.   Pour into the crock pot water, a sufficient amount to cover all the ingredients and about two inches more than that.

3.   Turn on the slow cooker to low and cook 6 hours, tasting and adding salt and pepper as needed.

4.   Serve hot and enjoy!

Nutritional Value:

Calories: 187;Carb: 5.4g ;Fat: 15.5g ;Protein: 21.4g

Ginger Beef with Peanut Sauce

Serves 4 Time: 8 hours on low

Ingredients:

- FOR THE STEAK
- ½ cup soy sauce or tamari
- 2 tablespoons water
- 2 tablespoons dry sherry or dry white wine
- 1 teaspoon blackstrap molasses
- 2 garlic cloves, minced
- 1 tablespoon minced fresh ginger
- 1½ teaspoons stevia powder
- 1 pound skirt steak, cubed
- 2 tablespoons toasted sesame oil
- FOR THE SAUCE
- ¾ cup coconut cream
- ½ cup all-natural peanut butter
- ½ cup water
- 2 tablespoons soy sauce or tamari
- 1 tablespoon freshly squeezed lime juice
- 1 garlic clove, minced
- 1 tablespoon erythritol or pinch stevia powder
- ½ teaspoon chili paste or red pepper flakes

Instructions:

TO MAKE THE STEAK

In the slow cooker, stir together the soy sauce, water, sherry, molasses, garlic, ginger, and stevia powder. Drizzle the steak with the sesame oil and add it to the slow cooker. Toss to coat the meat with the sauce. Cover and cook for 8 hours on low.

TO MAKE THE SAUCE: In a small saucepan set over medium heat, combine the coconut cream, peanut butter, water, soy sauce, lime juice, garlic, erythritol, and chili paste. Heat, stirring frequently, until the peanut butter melts and the sauce is a uniform consistency. Serve the meat hot, with the peanut sauce for dipping.

Nutrition Value: Calories: 625;Fat: 48g;Carbs: 12g;Protein: 38g

Onion Mushroom Cheesesteak Casserole

Serves 6

Time: 8 hours on low

Ingredients:

- 2 tablespoons coconut oil
- 1 onion, thinly sliced
- 8 ounces cremini or button mushrooms, sliced
- 1 green bell pepper, seeded and cut into strips
- 1 red bell pepper, seeded and cut into strips
- 1½ pounds rib eye steak
- ¾ teaspoon kosher salt
- ¾ teaspoon freshly ground black pepper
- 8 ounces provolone cheese, thinly sliced

Instructions:

1. In a large skillet, heat the coconut oil over medium-high heat. Add the onion and sauté until beginning to soften, about 3 minutes.

2. Add the mushrooms and continue to sauté until the mushrooms begin to brown, about 5 minutes. Transfer the mixture to the slow cooker.

3. Add the green and red bell peppers to the slow cooker and stir to mix.

4. Return the skillet to medium-high heat. Season the steak with the salt and pepper and add it to the skillet. Cook until browned, about 2 minutes per side. Transfer the steak to the slow cooker, placing it on top of the vegetables. Cover and cook for 8 hours on low.

5. Remove the steak from the cooker and let it rest for a couple of minutes. Leave the slow cooker on and keep it covered. After a few minutes, slice the steak into thin strips and return them to the slow cooker. Place the provolone cheese over the top, replace the cover, and let it sit for a few minutes until the cheese is melty. Serve hot.

Nutrition Value:

Calories: 734; Fat: 59g;Carbs: 8g;Protein: 43g

Tomato Sardines in Gravy

Serving: 8

Time: 7 hours

Ingredients

- 2 tablespoons olive oil
- 2 pound fresh sardines, cubed
- 4 plum tomatoes, chopped finely
- 1 large onion, sliced
- 2 garlic cloves, minced
- 1 cup homemade tomato puree
- Salt and freshly ground black pepper, to taste

Instructions:

1.   In a slow cooker, add oil in the bottom. Place sardine over oil. Top with remaining ingredients.

2.   Set the slow cooker on Low. Cover and cook for about 7 hours.

3.   Serve hot.

Nutrition Value:

Calories: 301

Fat: 16.7g

Carb: 7g

Protein: 9.4g

Yummy Onion Oregano Salmon Stew

Servings: 4

Time: 5 hours on high

Ingredients:

- 1 lb. salmon fillet, cubed
- 1 tbsp. coconut oil
- 1 medium onion, chopped
- 1 garlic clove, minced
- 1 sliced zucchini
- 1 seeded and cubed green bell pepper
- ½ cup chopped tomatoes
- 1 cup homemade fish broth
- ¼ tsp. dried and crushed oregano
- ¼ tsp. dried and crushed basil
- Salt
- Freshly ground black pepper

Instructions:

In a large slow cooker, add all ingredients and stir to combine.

Set the slow cooker on high. Cover and cook for about 5 hours.

Serve while hot.

Nutrition Value:

Calories: 223

Fat: 11g

Carb: 7g

Protein: 24.7g

Thyme Creamy Mushroom Chicken Soup

Serves 6

Time: 5.5 hours on low

Ingredients:

- 1 tablespoon coconut oil
- 10 ounces boneless, skinless chicken thighs, cut into 1-inch chunks
- Kosher salt
- Freshly ground black pepper
- 2 tablespoons unsalted butter
- 2 celery stalks, diced ½ onion, diced
- 3 garlic cloves, minced
- 8 ounces cremini mushrooms, thinly sliced
- 4 cups chicken broth, divided
- ½ teaspoon dried thyme
- 1 bay leaf
- 1 cup heavy (whipping) cream
- 2 tablespoons chopped fresh flat-leaf parsley

Instructions:

1. In a large skillet, heat the coconut oil over medium-high heat.

2. Season the chicken with salt and pepper and add it to the skillet. Sauté until browned on all sides, about 5 minutes. Transfer the chicken to the slow cooker.

3. Return the skillet to medium-high heat and add the butter. When it has melted, add the celery, onion, garlic, and mushrooms and sauté until softened, about 5 minutes.

4. Add 1 cup of chicken broth to the skillet to deglaze it. Bring to a boil and cook for about 1 minute, stirring and scraping up any browned bits from the bottom. Carefully pour the mixture into the slow cooker.

5. Stir the remaining 3 cups of broth, thyme, and bay leaf into the cooker. Cover and cook for 6 hours on low. Just before serving, stir in the heavy cream and parsley. Discard the bay leaf and serve hot.

Nutrition Value: Calories: 322; Fat: 25g;Carbs: 8g;Protein: 15g

Creamy Wine Sauce Garlic Shrimp

Serves: 4

Time: 2 hours

Ingredients

- 1 cup heavy whipping cream
- 1/2 cup grated parmesan cheese
- 1/2 cup dry white wine
- 4 garlic cloves, chopped finely
- 3 tbsp butter
- 1 lb shrimp, deveined

Instructions:

1.   Adjust the temperature to high. Sautee the garlic in the butter.

2.   When the garlic turn golden brown add the wine, the whipping cream, and the cheese.

3.   Put the lid on and cook 1 hour on low setting.

4.   Put the shrimp in.

5.   Cover and turn slow cooker to high. Cook for another hour.

6.   Serve.

Nutritional Value:

Calories: 390

Fat: 27.7g

Carb: 3.8g

Protein: 30.5g

Onion Balsamic Pot Roast

Time: 6 hours 10 minutes

Serving: 6

 Ingredients:

- 3 lbs chuck roast, boneless
- 1/2 cup tomato sauce
- 1/2 cup balsamic vinegar
- 1 cup beef stock
- 2 large onion, sliced
- 1/4 cup water
- 2 tbsp olive oil
- 1 tbsp steak rub
- Pepper

Instructions:

Rub steak seasoning and black pepper over meat.

Heat little olive oil in a pan over medium heat.

Place roast into the pan and cook until brown roast from both the sides.

Add beef stock into the saucepan and boil until sauce reduced to half then add tomato sauce and vinegar.

Add sliced onion into the slow cooker then place roast over the onions.

Pour beef stock mixture into the slow cooker.

Cover and cook on low for 6 hours. Serve warm and enjoy.

Nutritional Value

Calories 566 ;Fat 23.7 g;Carb: 6.5 g ;Protein 66.2 g

Ginger Coconut Lamb Curry

Serves 6

Time: 8 hours on low or 4 hours on high

Ingredients:

- 1½ pounds lamb stew meat, cut into 1½-inch cubes
- 1 onion, diced
- 2 garlic cloves, minced
- 1 tablespoon grated fresh ginger
- 1 tablespoon curry powder
- 1 teaspoon kosher salt
- ¾ teaspoon freshly ground black pepper
- ½ teaspoon cayenne pepper
- 1 (14-ounce) can coconut milk
- ¼ cup coconut oil, melted
- ½ cup ground toasted almonds (optional)
- 8 to 10 whole curry leaves or ½ cup chopped fresh cilantro

Instructions:

1. In the slow cooker, combine the lamb, onion, garlic, ginger, curry powder, salt, black pepper, and cayenne pepper.

2. Add the coconut milk and coconut oil and stir to mix. Cover and cook for 8 hours on low or 4 hours on high.

3. Serve hot, garnished with the ground almonds (if using) and curry leaves.

Nutrition Value:

Calories: 512

Fat: 44g

Carbs: 6g

Protein: 25g

Tamari Creamy Pork Loin

Serves 6

Time: 8 hours on low

Ingredients:

- 1 tablespoon kosher salt
- 2 teaspoons freshly ground black pepper
- 4 garlic cloves, minced
- 1 (3-pound) bone-in pork loin roast
- 2 onions, sliced
- ¼ cup water
- 2 tablespoons soy sauce or tamari
- 1 cup heavy (whipping) cream

Instructions:

1. In a small bowl, stir together the salt, pepper, and garlic to form a paste. Rub the seasoning mixture all over the pork roast.

2. Arrange the onions in the bottom of the slow cooker. Pour in the water and soy sauce. Place the roast on top of the onions. Cover and cook for 8 hours on low.

3. Remove the roast from the slow cooker and let it rest for 10 minutes.

4. While the roast is resting, transfer the remaining liquid and onions from the slow cooker to a blender. Add the heavy cream and process into a smooth sauce.

5. Slice the pork and serve it with the gravy spooned over the top.

Nutrition Value:

Calories: 524

Fat: 36g

Carbs: 6g

Protein: 44g

Rosemary Mushroom Chicken Cream

Serves 6

Time: 6 hours on low or 3 hours on high

Ingredients:

- 8 ounces bacon, diced
- 1½ pounds boneless, skinless chicken thighs
- ½ cup dry white wine
- ¼ cup (½ stick) unsalted butter, cubed
- 8 ounces cremini or button mushrooms, halved or quartered
- 1 onion, diced
- 6 garlic cloves, minced
- 3 fresh rosemary sprigs
- 1 teaspoon kosher salt
- 1 cup sour cream

Instructions:

1. In a large skillet, cook the bacon over medium-high heat until crisp, about 5 minutes. Transfer the bacon to the slow cooker.

2. Return the skillet to medium-high heat and add the chicken. Sauté until browned on both sides, about 4 minutes. Transfer the chicken to the slow cooker.

3. Add the wine to the skillet and bring to a boil. Cook for about 1 minute, stirring and scraping up any browned bits stuck to the bottom of the pan. Transfer to the slow cooker.

4. Add the butter, mushrooms, onion, garlic, rosemary, and salt to the slow cooker. Cover and cook for 6 hours on low or 3 hours on high.

5. Remove the chicken pieces and vegetables from the slow cooker and arrange them on a serving platter. Discard the rosemary sprigs. Stir the sour cream into the sauce in the cooker until well incorporated. Ladle the sauce over the chicken on the platter and serve hot.

Nutrition Value: Calories: 570; Fat: 49g;Carbs: 5g;Protein: 27g

Balsamic Olive Tomatoes Pot Roast

Time: 7 hours 20 minutes

Serving: 6

Ingredients:

- 3 lbs beef chuck roast
- 8 green olives, sliced
- 1 tsp arrowroot
- 1/4 Tsp black pepper
- 1 tsp Italian seasoning, dried
- 2 tbsp balsamic vinegar
- 1/2 cup dry red wine
- 1/4 cup sun-dried tomatoes, chopped
- 20 garlic cloves, peeled and sliced

Instructions:

Add sliced garlic and sun dried tomatoes into the slow cooker.

Place beef over the garlic and tomatoes.

Pour vinegar and red wine over meat.

Sprinkle with black pepper and Italian seasoning.

Cover and cook on low for 7 hours. Transfer meat on a platter.

Set slow cooker on high. In a small bowl, whisk together 2 tsp water and arrowroot and pour into the slow cooker. Stir well.

Cover and cook for another 10 minutes or until sauce thicken. Pour sauce over meat and stir in olives. Serve and enjoy.

Nutritional Value : Calories 870 ;Fat 62 g ;Carb: 5.1 g ;Protein 59 g

Parsley Garlic Butter Scallops

Serves: 3

Time: 1 hour

Ingredients

- 1 lb bay scallops
- 1 lemon, sliced
- 3 garlic cloves, halved
- 4 tablespoons butter
- 1/2 cup chopped parsley
- Salt and pepper as desired

Instructions:

1. Put the butter, lemon slices, salt, and pepper together on the bottom of the crock pot.
2. Put the lid on and adjust the temperature setting to high. Cook 30 min.
3. Add the pound of bay scallops, stirring.
4. Put the lid back on and cook for another 30 min.
5. Throw in the parsley last-minute.
6. Serve hot!

Nutritional Value:

Calories: 315

Fat: 16.7g

Carb: 8g

Protein: 31.7g

Lemon Parmesan Tilapia Fillet

Serving: 4

Time: 4 hours

Ingredients

- ½ cup Parmesan cheese, grated
- ¼ cup mayonnaise
- ¼ cup fresh lemon juice
- Salt and freshly ground black pepper, to taste
- 4 tilapia fillets
- 2 tablespoons fresh cilantro, chopped

Instructions:

1. In a bowl, mix together all ingredients except tilapia fillets and cilantro. Coat the fillets with mayonnaise mixture evenly. Place the filets onto a large foil paper. Wrap the foil paper around fillets to seal them. Arrange the foil packet in the bottom of a large slow cooker.

2. Set the slow cooker on Low. Cover and cook for 3-4 hours.

3. Serve with the garnishing of cilantro.

Nutritional Value:

Calories: 172

Fat: 11.1g

Carb: 4.6g

Protein: 13.3g

Lemon Turmeric Spinach Halibut

Serves: 4

Time: 2 hours

Ingredients

- Juice of 4 lemons
- 2 large halibut steaks
- 4 tbsp olive oil
- 1 tbsp cumin
- 1 tbsp turmeric
- 1/2 tsp cayenne pepper
- 4 cups fresh spinach
- 4 cloves minced garlic

Instructions:

1. Saute the garlic in the olive oil on the bottom on the high setting.
2. Add 2 tablespoons of water and the lemon juice.
3. Add the spices.
4. When everything has been stirred well, add the halibut steaks.
5. Cover and adjust the temperature to low.
6. Cook 2 hours.
7. Put in the spinach and stir well, allowing the spinach to cook in the residual heat. Serve.

Nutritional Value: Calories: 402;Fat: 30.6 g ;Carb: 7.8g ;Protein: 24.9g

Delicious Thyme Beef Roast

Time: 8 hours 10 minutes

Serving Size: 8

Ingredients:

- 2 1/2 lbs beef round roast
- 1/2 Tsp marjoram
- 1/2 Tsp thyme
- 1 tsp basil
- 1/2 cup red wine
- 1/2 cup water
- 1 small onion, sliced
- 1/4 Tsp pepper
- 1 tsp kosher salt

Instructions:

1. In a small bowl, combine together all spices. Set aside.
2. Place beef roast into the slow cooker.
3. Sprinkle spice mixture over roast and top with onion.
4. Pour water and wine into the slow cooker.
5. Cover and cook on low for 8 hours.
6. Once beef is cooked then using fork shred the meat. Serve and enjoy.

Nutritional Value

Calories 281

Fat 11 g

Carb: 1.3 g

Protein 39 g

Garlic Worcestershire Sauce Brisket

Time: 6 hours 30 minutes

Serving: 6

Ingredients:

- 3 1/2 lbs beef brisket
- 1 tbsp soy sauce
- 2 tbsp Worcestershire sauce
- 2 cups beef broth
- 2 large onion, sliced
- 1 tbsp olive oil
- 6 garlic cloves, minced
- Pepper
- Salt

Instructions:

Heat olive oil in the pan over medium heat.

Add onion into the pan and cook until lightly caramelized about 20 minutes.

Season brisket with pepper and salt. Heat another pan over medium heat.

Place brisket on the pan and cook until brisket appears golden brown crust.

Place brisket into the slow cooker. Sprinkle garlic over brisket then place caramelized onion over the brisket. Combine together soy sauce and Worcestershire sauce and pour over the brisket.

Cover slow cooker with lid and cook on low for 6 hours or until brisket is tender. Sliced brisket and serve.

Nutritional Value : Calories: 555 ;Fat: 19.4 g ;Carb: 7.2 g ;Protein 82.8 g

Chili Coconut Braised Short Ribs

Serves 6

Time: 9 hours on low or 4½ hours on high

Ingredients:

1 onion, diced

3 garlic cloves, minced

1 tablespoon minced fresh ginger

1 (14-ounce) can coconut milk

2 tablespoons soy sauce, tamari, or coconut aminos

2 tablespoons mirin

2 tablespoons toasted sesame oil

2 teaspoons blackstrap molasses

1 teaspoon or less chili paste for seasoning

1 teaspoon stevia powder

1 pound short ribs

3 scallions, thinly sliced

¼ cup toasted sesame seeds

Instructions:

1. In the slow cooker, stir together the onion, garlic, ginger, coconut milk, soy sauce, mirin, sesame oil, molasses, chili paste, and stevia powder.

2. Add the short ribs and stir to coat them well. Cover and cook for 9 hours on low or 4½ hours on high. Serve hot, garnished with the scallions and sesame seeds.

Nutrition Value: Calories: 553; Fat: 50g;Carbs: 12g;Protein: 16g

KETO SLOW COOKER DINNER RECIPES

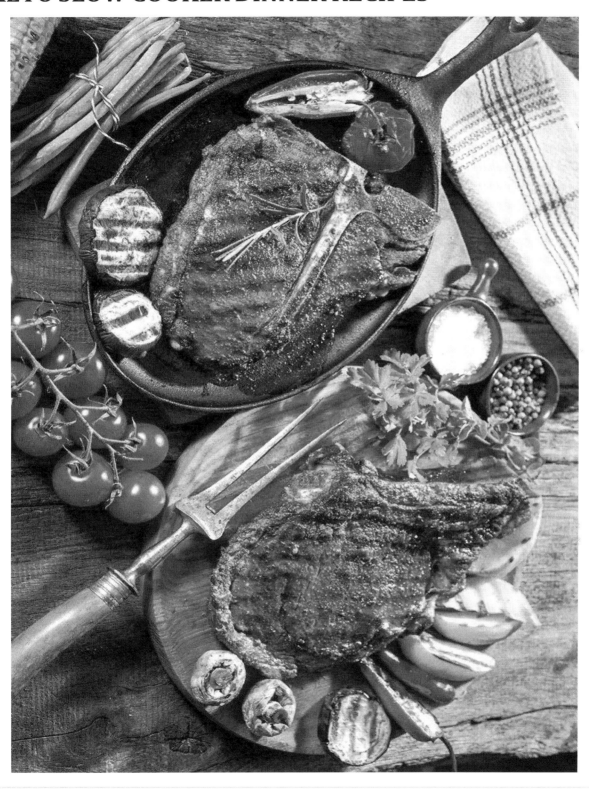

Yogurt Turkey Meatballs

Serves 6
Time: 7 hours on low
Ingredients:

- FOR THE MEATBALLS
- 1¼ pounds ground turkey
- 1 cup crumbled feta cheese
- ½ cup finely chopped walnuts
- ½ cup minced fresh mint
- ¼ cup grated onion
- 4 garlic cloves, minced
- 3 tablespoons paprika
- 1 tablespoon ground cumin
- 1½ teaspoons kosher salt
- 1 teaspoon freshly ground black pepper
- ¼ to ½ teaspoon cayenne pepper
- 2 tablespoons extra-virgin olive oil
- 1 onion, halved and thinly sliced
- 1 cup chicken broth

TO MAKE THE MEATBALLS

1. In a large bowl, stir together the ground turkey, feta, walnuts, mint, onion, garlic, paprika, cumin, salt, black pepper, and cayenne pepper. Form the mixture into about 24 oblong meatballs.
2. In the slow cooker insert, combine the olive oil and onion and spread to cover the bottom of the cooker. Top with the meatballs.
3. Pour in the chicken broth. Cover and cook for 7 hours on low.

FOR THE SAUCE

1 cup plain full-fat Greek yogurt
2 tablespoons tahini
1 tablespoon freshly squeezed lemon juice
½ teaspoon kosher salt
1 tablespoon extra-virgin olive oil
1 teaspoon za'atar (optional)
½ teaspoon ground sumac (optional)

TO MAKE THE SAUCE

1. In a small bowl, whisk together the yogurt, tahini, lemon juice, and salt.
2. Garnish the sauce with a drizzle of olive oil and a sprinkling of za'atar and sumac (if using). Serve the meatballs hot, with the sauce alongside for dipping.

Nutrition Value:

Calories: 443, Fat: 35g, Carbs: 9g, Protein: 25g

Parsley Wine Tomato-braised Tuna

Serving: 8

Ingredients:

- 2 tuna fillets (3 pounds)
- ½ cup olive oil
- 1 small red onion, chopped
- 6 cloves garlic, minced
- 3 cups gluten free, sugar-free tomato sauce
- 1 cup dry white wine
- 6 tablespoons drained and rinsed capers
- 4 tablespoons chopped fresh parsley
- 2 bay leaves
- Sea salt
- Freshly ground black pepper

Instructions:

Place the tuna in a bowl of cold salted water to soak for about 12 minutes. Drain well and pat dry using paper towels.

Place a skillet over medium high flame and heat 2 tablespoons of oil. Sauté the onion and garlic until the onion is translucent. Transfer into the slow cooker.

Stir the wine, tomato, or marinara sauce, capers, bay leaves, and parsley into the slow cooker. Cover and cook for 1 hour on high.

Place the skillet over medium high heat and heat the rest of the oil. Brown the tuna fillets all over, then place into the slow cooker.

Cover and cook for 1 hour and 30 minutes on high, or until the tuna is cooked.

Nutrition Value: Calories: 155; Fat: 16.5g;Carbs: 8g; Protein: 40g

Garlic Cabbage Beef Soup

Serves 6

Time: 8 to 10 hours on low

Ingredients:

- 2 tablespoons coconut oil
- 8 ounces beef stew meat, diced
- Kosher salt
- Freshly ground black pepper
- 8 ounces smoked beef sausage, diced
- 1 onion, finely chopped
- 3 cups shredded cabbage
- 2 cups beef broth
- 1 (15-ounce) can tomato sauce
- 2 garlic cloves, minced
- 2 bay leaves
- 3 tablespoons chopped fresh parsley
- 1 cup sour cream

Instructions:

1. In a large skillet, heat the coconut oil over medium-high heat.

2. Generously season the meat with salt and pepper and add it to the skillet, along with the sausage. Cook until the meat is browned on all sides, about 6 minutes. Transfer the beef and sausage to the slow cooker.

3. Return the skillet to medium-high heat and add the onion. Sauté until softened, about 4 minutes. Transfer the onion to the slow cooker.

4. Add the cabbage, beef broth, tomato sauce, garlic, and bay leaves to the slow cooker. Cover and cook for 8 to 10 hours on low.

5. Discard the bay leaves and serve hot, garnished with the parsley and a dollop of sour cream.

Nutrition Value: Calories: 329;Fat: 26g;Carbs: 9g;Protein: 16g

Mushrooms & Bell Pepper Cheesesteak

Serves 6

Time: 8 hours on low

Ingredients:

- 2 tablespoons coconut oil
- 1 onion, thinly sliced
- 8 ounces cremini or button mushrooms, sliced
- 1 green bell pepper, seeded and cut into strips
- 1 red bell pepper, seeded and cut into strips
- 1½ pounds rib eye steak
- ¾ teaspoon kosher salt
- ¾ teaspoon freshly ground black pepper
- 8 ounces provolone cheese, thinly sliced

Instructions:

1. In a large skillet, heat the coconut oil over medium-high heat. Add the onion and sauté until beginning to soften, about 3 minutes.

2. Add the mushrooms and continue to sauté until the mushrooms begin to brown, about 5 minutes. Transfer the mixture to the slow cooker.

3. Add the green and red bell peppers to the slow cooker and stir to mix.

4. Return the skillet to medium-high heat. Season the steak with the salt and pepper and add it to the skillet. Cook until browned, about 2 minutes per side. Transfer the steak to the slow cooker, placing it on top of the vegetables. Cover and cook for 8 hours on low.

5. Remove the steak from the cooker and let it rest for a couple of minutes. Leave the slow cooker on and keep it covered. After a few minutes, slice the steak into thin strips and return them to the slow cooker. Place the provolone cheese over the top, replace the cover, and let it sit for a few minutes until the cheese is melty. Serve hot.

Nutrition Value:

Calories: 734

Fat: 59g

Carbs: 8g

Protein: 43g

Lemon Garlic Shrimp Scampi

Serves: 6

Time: 1.5 hours

Ingredients

- 1 lb raw shrimp, peeled and deveined
- Juice of one fresh lemon
- 1/2 cup chicken broth
- 3 cloves minced garlic
- 4 tbsp butter
- 2 tbsp fresh parsley
- Salt and pepper as desired

Instructions:

1. Adjust the heat of the slow cooker to high.

2. Combine the chicken broth, lemon juice, butter, garlic, parsley, salt, and pepper in the crockpot. Stir thoroughly.

3. Put the shrimp in, mixing well.

4. Put the lid on

5. Cook 1.5 hours.

6. Serve.

Nutritional Value:

Calories: 250

Fat: 13.7 g

Carb: 4.6g

Protein: 27g

Delicious Curry Beef

Serves 6

Time: 8 hours on low

Ingredients:

- 1 cup diced tomatoes
- 1 (14-ounce) can coconut milk
- ⅓ cup water
- ¼ cup coconut oil, melted
- ¼ cup tomato paste
- 1 onion, diced
- 6 garlic cloves, minced
- 3 tablespoons grated fresh ginger
- 2 tablespoons ground cumin
- 1 teaspoon paprika
- 1 teaspoon kosher salt
- ½ teaspoon ground turmeric
- ½ teaspoon ground cardamom
- ½ teaspoon ground cinnamon
- ½ teaspoon ground cloves
- ½ teaspoon cayenne pepper
- ¼ teaspoon ground nutmeg
- 1 (1½-pound) beef chuck roast, cut into ½-by-2-inch strips
- ⅓ cup chopped fresh cilantro

Instructions:

1. In the slow cooker, stir together the tomatoes, coconut milk, water, coconut oil, and tomato paste.

2. Add the onion, garlic, ginger, cumin, paprika, salt, turmeric, cardamom, cinnamon, cloves, cayenne, and nutmeg.

3. Add the beef and toss to mix well. Cover and cook for 8 hours on low. Serve hot, garnished with the cilantro.

Nutrition Value:

Calories: 547

Fat: 46g

Carbs: 12g

Protein: 26g

Heavy Creamy Herb Pork Chops

Serves 4

Time: 8 hours on low or 4 hours on high

Ingredients:

- ¾ cup chicken or beef broth
- 2 tablespoons coconut oil, melted
- 1 tablespoon Dijon mustard
- 2 garlic cloves, minced
- 1 tablespoon paprika
- 1 tablespoon onion powder
- 1 teaspoon dried oregano
- 1 teaspoon dried basil
- 1 teaspoon dried parsley
- 1 onion, thinly sliced
- 4 thick-cut boneless pork chops
- 1 cup heavy (whipping) cream

Instructions:

1. In the slow cooker, stir together the broth, coconut oil, mustard, garlic, paprika, onion powder, oregano, basil, and parsley.

2. Add the onion and pork chops and toss to coat. Cover and cook for 8 hours on low or 4 hours on high.

3. Transfer the chops to a serving platter. Transfer the remaining juices and onion in the slow cooker to a blender, add the heavy cream, and process until smooth. Pour the sauce over the pork chops and serve hot.

Nutrition Value:

Calories: 470

Fat: 32g

Carbs: 7g

Protein: 39g

Mushroom Beef Stroganoff

Serves 6

Time: 8 hours on low

Ingredients:

- 2 pounds beef stew meat, cut into 1-inch cubes
- 4 bacon slices, diced
- 8 ounces cremini or button mushrooms, quartered
- 1 onion, halved and sliced
- 2 garlic cloves, minced
- 1 cup beef broth
- ¼ cup tomato paste
- 1 teaspoon smoked paprika
- ½ teaspoon kosher salt
- ¼ teaspoon freshly ground black pepper
- 1½ cups sour cream
- 2 tablespoons minced fresh parsley

Instructions:

1. In the slow cooker, stir together the beef, bacon, mushrooms, onion, garlic, beef broth, tomato paste, paprika, salt, and pepper. Cover and cook for 8 hours on low.

2. Just before serving, stir in the sour cream. Serve hot, garnished with the parsley.

Nutrition Value:

Calories: 594

Fat: 47g

Carb: 7g

Protein: 35g

Ginger Cream Sauce Pork Loin

Serves 6
Time: 8 hours on low
Ingredients:

- FOR THE PORK
- 1 tablespoon erythritol
- 2 teaspoons kosher salt
- 1 teaspoon garlic powder
- 1 teaspoon ground ginger
- ½ teaspoon ground cinnamon
- ½ teaspoon ground cloves
- ½ teaspoon red pepper flakes
- ¼ teaspoon freshly ground black pepper
- 1 (2-pound) pork shoulder roast
- ½ cup water

TO MAKE THE PORK

1. In a small bowl, stir together the erythritol, salt, garlic powder, ginger, cinnamon, cloves, red pepper flakes, and black pepper. Rub the seasoning mixture all over the pork and place it in the slow cooker.
2. Pour the water into the cooker around the pork. Cover and cook for 8 hours on low.
3. Remove the pork from the slow cooker and let it rest for about 5 minutes.

FOR THE SAUCE

2 tablespoons unsalted butter
3 tablespoons minced fresh ginger
2 shallots, minced
1 tablespoon minced garlic
⅔ cup dry white wine
1 cup heavy (whipping) cream

TO MAKE THE SAUCE

1. While the pork rests, melt the butter in a small saucepan over medium heat.
2. Stir in the ginger, shallots, and garlic.
3. Add the white wine and bring to a boil. Cook, stirring, until the liquid is reduced to about ¼ cup, about 5 minutes.
4. Whisk in the heavy cream and continue to boil, stirring, until the sauce thickens, 3 to 5 minutes more.
5. Slice the pork and serve it with the sauce spooned over the top.

Nutrition Value:
Calories: 488
Fat: 40g
Carb: 5g
Protein: 27g

Heavy Cream Chicken Stew

Serves 4

Time: 7 hours on low

Ingredients:

- ¼ cup extra-virgin olive oil
- 12 ounces whole chicken legs and thighs
- 1 cup chicken broth
- 1 cup pitted green or black olives
- 1 stalk celery, chopped
- ½ onion, diced
- 2 garlic cloves, minced
- 2 tablespoons dry white wine
- 1 tablespoon tomato paste
- 1 teaspoon fennel seeds, crushed
- ½ teaspoon kosher salt
- 1 cup heavy (whipping) cream
- 2 tablespoons chopped fresh parsley

Instructions:

1. In the slow cooker, combine the olive oil, chicken, chicken broth, olives, celery, onion, garlic, white wine, tomato paste, fennel seeds, and salt. Stir to mix. Cover and cook for 7 hours on low.

2. Just before serving, stir in the heavy cream and the parsley.

Nutrition Value:

Calories: 447

Fat: 34g

Carbs: 7g

Protein: 26g

Toasted Almond Braised Beef

Serves 4 to 6

Time: 9 hours on low or 4½ hours on high

Ingredients:

- ¼ cup coconut oil
- 1 medium onion, diced
- 2 teaspoons ground cumin
- 1½ teaspoons kosher salt
- ½ teaspoon freshly ground black pepper
- ½ teaspoon ground cinnamon
- ½ teaspoon ground ginger
- 1 cup dry red wine
- 1 (1¼-pound) beef chuck roast, cut into 2-inch pieces
- Grated zest and juice of 1 orange
- 1 cup heavy (whipping) cream
- 5 tablespoons unsalted butter
- ½ cup ground toasted almonds
- ¼ cup chopped fresh cilantro

Instructions:

1. In a large skillet, heat the coconut oil over medium-high heat. Add the onion and sauté until soft, about 5 minutes.

2. Add the cumin, salt, pepper, cinnamon, and ginger. Sauté for 1 minute more.

3. Stir in the red wine and bring to a boil. Cook for 1 to 2 minutes, scraping up any browned bits from the bottom of the pan. Transfer the mixture to the slow cooker.

4. Stir in the beef, orange zest, and orange juice. Cover and cook for 9 hours on low or 4½ hours on high.

5. Stir in the heavy cream and butter until the butter melts and both are well incorporated. Serve hot, garnished with the almonds and cilantro.

Nutrition Value:

Calories: 747

Fat: 56g

Carbs: 9g

Protein: 47g

Coconut Pumpkin Pork Stew

Serves 8

Time: 8 hours on low

Ingredients:

- 2 tablespoons coconut oil
- 1½ pounds boneless pork ribs
- Kosher salt
- Freshly ground black pepper
- ½ onion, chopped
- 1 garlic clove, minced
- 1 jalapeño pepper, seeded and minced
- 1 teaspoon minced fresh ginger
- 1½ cups chicken broth
- 3 cups canned coconut milk
- 1 cup pumpkin purée
- ¼ cup all-natural peanut butter
- ¼ cup erythritol
- 1 teaspoon freshly squeezed lime juice
- ¼ cup chopped fresh cilantro
- ½ cup chopped toasted peanuts

Instructions:

1. In a large skillet, heat the coconut oil over medium-high heat.

2. Generously season the pork with salt and pepper and add it to the skillet. Cook until browned on both sides, about 6 minutes. Transfer to the slow cooker.

3. Return the skillet to medium-high heat and add the onion, garlic, jalapeño, and ginger. Sauté until the onions are softened, about 3 minutes.

4. Stir in the chicken broth and bring to a boil. Cook for 1 minute.

5. Stir in the coconut milk, pumpkin, peanut butter, and erythritol until smooth. Pour the mixture into the slow cooker. Cover and cook for 8 hours on low.

6. Remove the meat from the slow cooker and cut it into bite-size pieces or shred it using two forks. Return the meat to the cooker.

7. Stir in the lime juice. Serve hot, garnished with the cilantro and peanuts.

Nutrition Value: Calories: 492; Fat: 41g; Carb: 11g; Protein: 24g

Ginger Spinach Chicken

Serves: 8

Time: 5 hours

Ingredients

- 1/2 cup liquid aminos
- 1 tbsp fresh ginger, minced
- 8 chicken thighs
- 2 cups water
- 1 tbsp garlic powder
- 1 tsp blackstrap molasses
- Salt and pepper to taste
- 2 cups spinach, whole leaves

Instructions:

1. Mix together the water and liquid aminos.
2. Put this mixture in the crockpot
3. Add all the other spices and mix this in thoroughly as well.
4. Place the chicken thighs in the liquid in the slow cooker.
5. Adjust the heat setting to high heat and put the lid on.
6. Allow to cook for 5 hours.
7. Add the spinach to the mixture in the crockpot.
8. Recover and cook on high for ten minutes, stirring occasionally.
9. Serve hot.

Nutrition Value:

Calories: 472

Fat: 35.7g

Carb:3.8g

Protein: 32.7g

Ghee Salmon with Fresh Cucumber Salad

Serves: 8

Time: 3 hours

Ingredients:

- 4 x 4oz Wild salmon fillets
- 2 tsp Tandoori spice
- 1 tsp salt
- 1 tsp black pepper
- 4 tbsp ghee
- Cucumber Salad
- 1 English cucumber
- 1 cup arugula
- ½ cup parsley
- ¼ cup lemon juice
- 2 tbsp extra virgin olive oil

Instructions:

1. Heat ghee in skillet over medium heat along with tandoori spice for a minute.

2. Place salmon filets in slow cooker, skin side down, sprinkle with salt, black pepper, and pour Tandoori butter over salmon.

3. Cook on high for 3.5 hours.

4. While salmon is cooking, dice cucumber, and toss with arugula, parsley, lemon juice and extra virgin olive oil.

5. Serve salmon with fresh cucumber salad.

Nutrition Value

Calories 413

Carbs 4 g

Fat 34 g

Protein 25 g

Delicious Short Ribs

Serves: 8

Time: 4 hours

Ingredients:

- 4 lbs short ribs, bone in
- 8 peppercorns
- 2 cups low-sodium beef
- 1 onion, diced
- 2 carrots, peeled, diced
- 2 celery stalks, diced
- 4 cloves, minced
- 1 tsp thyme
- 1 tsp rosemary
- 2 bay leaves
- 2 tsp salt
- 2 tsp black pepper
- Extra virgin olive oil

Instructions:

1.   Heat 4 tbsp extra virgin olive oil in skillet. Add onions and garlic, and sauté until brown.

2.   Place onion mixture in slow cooker, add short ribs along with carrots, celery stalk, cloves, thyme, rosemary, peppercorns, bay leaves, salt, and black pepper.

3.   Cook on high for 4 hours.

Nutrition Value:

Calories 520

Fat: 24g

Carbs 3.7 g

Protein 67 g

Cilantro Chili Verde

Serves: 8

Time: 7 hours

Ingredients:

- 1½ lbs pork shoulder
- ½ lb sirloin, cubed
- 4 Anaheim chilies, stemmed
- 6 cloves garlic, minced
- ½ cup cilantro, chopped
- 2 onions, peeled and sliced
- 2 tomatoes, chopped.
- 1 tbsp tomato paste
- 1 lime
- 1 tbsp cumin
- 1 tbsp oregano
- Extra virgin olive oil

Instructions:

1. Slice pork shoulder into ½" cubes, and set slow cooker to medium.

2. Heat 4 tbsp extra virgin olive oil in skillet, add onions, Anaheim chilies, and garlic, and sauté for 2 minutes.

3. Place skillet mixture into slow cooker, add pork shoulder, sirloin, and stir.

4. Add tomatoes, cilantro, tomato paste, cumin, oregano, and salt to pot.

5. Cover and cook for 7 hours.

6. Squeeze a little of lime in each bowl when serving.

Nutrition Value

Calories 262

Fat 16 g

Carbs 6 g

Protein 23 g

Ginger Coconut Chicken Wings

Serving: 6

Time: 6 hours 10 minutes

Ingredients:

- 3 lbs chicken wings
- 1 tbsp fresh cilantro, minced
- 1 tbsp fresh ginger, minced
- 1 tbsp coconut milk
- 2 oz Thai basil, minced
- 8 oz green curry paste

Instructions:

Add chicken wings into the slow cooker.

In a bowl, whisk together coconut milk, cilantro, ginger, basil, and curry paste.

Pour coconut milk mixture over chicken wings and toss well.

Cover and cook on low for 6 hours.

Stir well and serve.

Nutritional Value

Calories: 322

Fat: 14.3 g

Carb: 6.3 g

Protein 39.6 g

Pepper Flakes Smoked Garlic Shrimp

Serving : 8

Time: 1 hour

Ingredients:

- 2 lbs raw shrimp, peeled and deveined
- 1/4 Tsp red pepper flakes, crushed
- 1/4 Tsp ground black pepper
- 1 tsp paprika
- 6 garlic cloves, sliced
- 3/4 cup olive oil
- 1 tsp kosher salt

Instructions:

Combine together oil, red pepper flakes, black pepper, paprika, garlic, and salt into the slow cooker.

Cover and cook on high for 30 minutes.

Add shrimp and stir well.

Cover and cook on high for 10 minutes.

Open the lid and stir again. Cover and cook for another 10 minutes.

Serve warm and enjoy.

Nutrition Value

Calories: 301

Fat :20 g

Carb: 2.7 g

Protein 26 g

Savory Onion Bacon Pork Chops

Serves: 4

Time: 3 hours

Ingredients

- 4 pieces of bacon sliced thinly
- 1 large diced onion
- 2 cups chicken broth
- 3 cloves garlic thick sliced
- 1 tbsp Worcestershire sauce
- 4 thick pork chops, bone-in
- 2 tbsp apple cider vinegar
- Salt and pepper as desired

Instructions:

1. Adjust the temperature to high heat and begin to cook the bacon on the bottom of it.

2. Once the bacon is giving off grease, put in the garlic and onions and cook them until golden.

3. Rub the pork chops all over with salt and pepper.

4. Put them in the slow cooker them with the onions, garlic, and bacon.

5. Pour the apple cider vinegar, Worcestershire sauce, and chicken broth.

6. Adjust the temperature to medium heat and put the lid on the crockpot.

7. Cook for three hours.

8. Serve.

Nutritional Values:

Calories: 467

Fat: 28g

Carb: 6.5g

Protein: 45g

Healthy Vegetable Beef Stew

Serves: 4-5

Ingredients:

- 1 ¼ pounds beef braising, boneless, pat dried
- ½ cup vegetable broth or water
- 2 cloves garlic, peeled
- 1.1 pounds zucchini or marrow squash, diced
- ½ teaspoon ground ginger
- 1 tablespoon ground cumin
- ½ teaspoon ground coriander
- ½ tablespoon paprika
- ½ teaspoon chili powder
- ½ teaspoon turmeric powder
- 2 small onions, chopped
- 1 bay leaf
- Salt and freshly ground pepper to taste
- 1 teaspoon dried rosemary, crushed
- 1 stick cinnamon
- ¼ cup ghee or lard or tallow
- 7 ounces canned chopped tomatoes
- A handful parsley, chopped to garnish

Instructions:

1. Set the slow cooker on 'High' and preheat.
2. Sprinkle salt and pepper on the steaks.
3. Place a skillet over medium heat. Add a little ghee. Add 2 steaks and sauté until brown. Cook in batches. Remove with a slotted spoon and transfer to the slow cooker.
4. Add more ghee if required. Add onion and garlic and sauté until light brown. Add rest of the ingredients except zucchini and rutabaga and stir for a couple of minutes.
5. Transfer into the slow cooker. Stir well.
6. Close the lid. Set cooker on 'High' option and timer for 2 ½ hours.
7. Move the meat to one side of the slow cooker. Add rutabaga to the other side. Cover and cook for an hour. Discard bay leaf and cinnamon stick.
8. Place zucchini along with the rutabaga. Mix it lightly with the cooking liquid but do not mix the meat part. Cook for 1 ½ hours or until the vegetables are tender.
9. Serve in bowls. Garnish with parsley and serve.

Nutritional value:

Calories: 533
Fat: 39.5g
Carb: 12g
Protein: 31.9g

Creamy Spicy Coconut Chicken

Serving Size: 5

Time: 6 hours 10 minutes

Ingredients:

- 1 lb chicken thighs, boneless and skinless
- 1 cup coconut milk
- 1 cup heavy cream
- 10 oz tomatoes, diced
- 2 tsp paprika
- 5 tsp garam masala
- 3 tbsp tomato paste
- 1 tbsp ginger, grated
- 3 garlic cloves, minced
- 2 tsp onion powder
- 2 tbsp olive oil
- 1 tsp guar gum

Instructions:

Cut chicken into the pieces and add in the slow cooker.

Add grated ginger over the chicken then add all spices.

Add tomatoes, tomato paste, and olive oil. Mix well.

Add half cup coconut milk and stir well. Cover slow cooker with lid and cook on low for 6 hours.

Once the chicken is cooked then add heavy cream, guar gum, and remaining coconut milk and stir well. Serve and enjoy.

Nutritional Value:

Calories: 444

Fat 33 g

Carb: 10 g

Protein 29.2 g

Garlic Jalapeno Curry Chicken Meatballs

Serves: 3

Ingredients:

- 1 pound 95% lean ground chicken
- 1 tablespoon fresh cilantro, chopped
- 2 green onions, chopped
- 1 tablespoon fresh ginger, minced, divided
- 2 cloves garlic, minced, divided
- 2 tablespoons Thai green curry paste, divided or more to taste
- 1 cup light coconut milk
- 1 jalapeño, sliced (optional)
- 2 tablespoons almond meal
- 1 tablespoon fresh basil, chopped
- Salt to taste
- Pepper to taste
- ½ cup chicken broth

Instructions:

1. Add chicken, green onion, almond meal, cilantro, basil, half the ginger, garlic and Thai curry paste, salt, and pepper into a bowl and mix well.

2. Divide the mixture into 12 equal portions and shape into balls.

3. Add rest of the ingredients into the slow cooker and mix well. Lower the balls into the slow cooker.

4. Close the lid. Set cooker on 'Low' option and timer for 3-4 hours or on 'High' option and timer for 1 ½ -2 hours.

Nutritional value:

Calories: 284

Fat :15 g

Carb: 3g

Protein: 33 g

Delight Foil Wrapped Fish

Serves: 3

Ingredients:

- 3 fish fillets of your choice
- Salt to taste
- Pepper to taste
- Any other seasoning of your choice

Instructions:

1. Take 3 large sheets of foil
2. Season the fillets with salt, pepper, and seasoning. Place a fillet on each foil.
3. Wrap each into a packet. Place the foil packets in the slow cooker.
4. Close the lid. Set cooker on 'Low' option and timer for 2-3 hours or on 'High' option and timer for 1-1 ½ hours.
5. Unwrap and serve.

Nutritional value:

Calories: 156

Fat : 9.2 g

Carb: 0g

Protein: 16.9 g

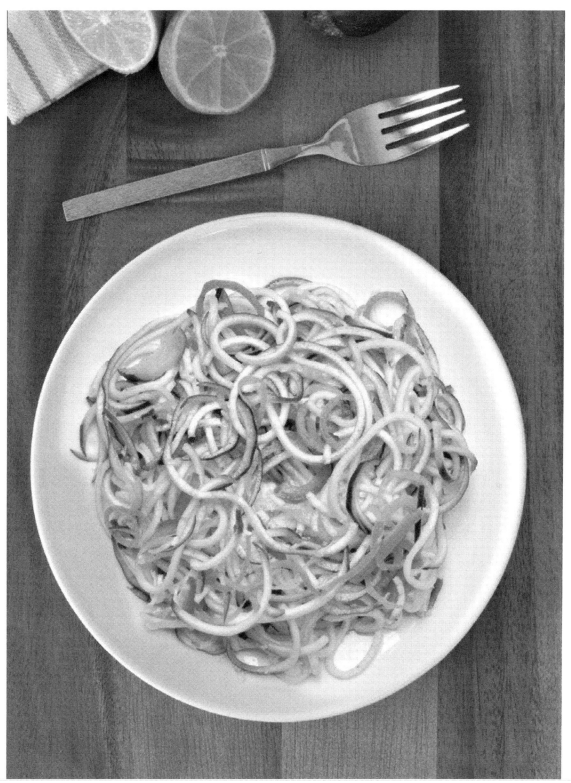

Cheddar Vegetarian Chili

Serves 8

Time: 7 hours on low or 4 hours on high

Ingredients:

- ¼ cup coconut oil
- 1 pound firm tofu, diced
- 1 (14.5-ounce) can diced tomatoes, with juice
- 1 onion, diced
- 3 garlic cloves, minced
- 1 or 2 jalapeño peppers, seeded and minced
- 3 tablespoons unsweetened cocoa powder
- 2 tablespoons chili powder
- 1½ teaspoons paprika
- 1½ teaspoons ground cumin
- 1 teaspoon ground cinnamon
- 1 teaspoon kosher salt
- ½ teaspoon dried oregano
- 2½ cups sour cream, divided
- 2 cups shredded Cheddar cheese
- 1 avocado, peeled, pitted, and sliced

Instructions:

1. In the slow cooker, combine the coconut oil, tofu, tomatoes and their juice, onion, garlic, jalapeños, cocoa powder, chili powder, paprika, cumin, cinnamon, salt, and oregano. Cover and cook for 8 hours on low or 4 hours on high.

2. Just before serving, stir in 1½ cups of sour cream. Serve hot, garnished with the remaining 1 cup of sour cream, Cheddar cheese, and avocado.

Nutrition Value:

Calories: 392

Fat: 34g

Carbs: 9g

Protein: 15g

Thyme Oregano Garlic Mushrooms

Serving: 4

Time: 3-4 hours on low

Ingredients:

- 24 ounces cremini mushrooms
- 4 minced garlic cloves
- ½ tsp. basil, dried
- ½ tsp. oregano, dried
- ¼ tsp. dried thyme
- 2 bay leaves
- 1 cup vegetable broth
- ¼ cup Half-and-half
- 2 tbsps. unsalted butter
- 2 tbsps. freshly chopped parsley leaves
- Kosher sea salt
- Black pepper

Instructions:

Combine all the ingredients except the butter, half and half and fresh parsley in a slow cooker.

Cook covered for 3-4 hours on low.

20 minutes prior to the completion of cook time, mix in the butter and half-and-half.

Garnish with parsley and serve.

Nutrition Value:

Calories: 120

Fat: 9g

Carbs: 6g

Protein: 6g

Ricotta Spinach Zucchini Lasagna

Serving: 8

Time: 3½ - 4 hours on high

Ingredients:

- 4 sliced zucchini
- 4 cups of homemade tomato sauce
- 15 ounces ricotta cheese
- 1 large egg
- ¼ cup freshly grated Parmesan cheese
- 1 cup chopped spinach
- Salt
- Pepper
- 16 ounces shredded mozzarella
- 2 tsps. freshly chopped parsley

Instructions:

Mix together the spinach, egg, ricotta cheese and half the Parmesan cheese in a bowl.

Spread a cup of tomato sauce in a greased slow cooker and spread 5 zucchini slices over it, slightly overlapping.

Spread some of the egg mixture over and sprinkle some Mozzarella.

Repeat the layering until all the ingredients are used up, topping with Parmesan cheese and Mozzarella.

Cook covered for 3½ - 4 hours on high. Serve garnished with parsley.

Nutritional Value:

Calories: 251

Fat: 14g

Carbs: 11g

Protein: 20.8g

Cheesy Spinach Stuffed Mushrooms

Serves 6

Time: 6 hours on low

Ingredients:

- 2 tablespoons unsalted butter, Ghee or extra-virgin olive oil
- 3 large eggs
- 2 cups shredded Gruyère cheese, divided
- ½ cup chopped walnuts, plus more for garnish
- 1½ pounds cremini or button mushrooms, stems minced, caps left whole
- 2 cups chopped spinach
- ½ onion, minced
- 2 garlic cloves, minced
- 1 tablespoon fresh thyme leaves, plus more for garnish
- ½ teaspoon kosher salt
- ½ teaspoon freshly ground black pepper

Instructions:

1. Generously coat the inside of the slow cooker insert with the butter.

2. In a medium bowl, beat the eggs, then stir in 1½ cups of Gruyère cheese, ½ cup of walnuts, the mushroom stems, spinach, onion, garlic, 1 tablespoon of thyme, salt, and pepper.

3. Spoon the mixture into the mushroom caps and place each filled cap in the bottom of the slow cooker in a single layer.

4. Sprinkle the remaining ½ cup of Gruyère cheese over the top. Cover and cook for 6 hours on low. Serve hot, garnished with additional thyme and chopped walnuts.

Nutrition Value

Calories: 382

Fat: 31g

Carbs: 9g

Protein: 20g

Rosemary Cheesy Broccoli

Serving: 10

Time: 5-6 hours

Ingredients:

- 8 cups broccoli florets
- 1 large onion, chopped
- 1 tablespoon fresh rosemary, minced
- 1½ cups Swiss cheese, grated
- 1¾ cups homemade tomato sauce
- 1 tbsp. fresh lemon juice
- Sea salt and freshly ground black pepper

Instructions:

In a large slow cooker, place all ingredients and mix well.

Set the slow cooker on Low. Cover and cook for about 5-6 hours. Serve hot.

Nutrition Value:

Calories: 104

Fat: 9g

Carbs: 5g

Protein: 7.2g

Garlic Spinach Curry

Serving: 8

Time: 3-4 hours on low

Ingredients:

- 3 packages (10 ounces) frozen spinach (thawed)
- 1 chopped onion
- 4 minced garlic cloves
- 2 tbsps. curry powder
- 2 tbsps. melted butter
- ½ cup vegetable stock
- ¼ cup heavy cream
- 1 tsp. lemon juice

Instructions:

Dump all ingredients in a crock pot except the cream and lemon juice.

Cook covered for 3-4 hours on low.

Mix in the lemon juice and cream, 30 minutes prior to the completion of cook time and cook covered. Serve warm.

Nutrition Value:

Calories: 91

Fat: 7g

Carbs: 3g

Protein: 4g

Parmesan Veggie Casserole

Serving: 10

Time: 3 hours

Ingredients:

- 1 tbsp. unsalted butter, melted
- 4 medium zucchinis, peeled and sliced
- 1 green bell pepper, seeded and sliced
- 2 cups finely chopped fresh tomatoes
- 1 thinly sliced white onion
- 1 tbsp. fresh thyme, minced
- ½ cup grated Parmesan cheese
- Sea salt
- Freshly ground black pepper

Instructions:

In a large slow cooker, place all ingredients except cheese and mix well.

Set the slow cooker on low. Cover and cook for about 3 hours.

Uncover and sprinkle with cheese evenly. Cover and cook for about 1½ hours.

Serve hot.

Nutritional Value:

Calories: 90

Fat: 8g

Carbs: 5g

Protein: 6g

Parmesan Tomato Eggplant

Serves 6

Time: 7 hours on low or 4 hours on high

Ingredients:

- 2 tablespoons coconut oil
- 2 cups tomato sauce
- 8 ounces mascarpone cheese
- 8 ounces eggplant, peeled and thinly sliced
- 3 cups shredded fontina cheese
- 1 cup grated Parmesan cheese
- 1 cup coarsely ground almond meal

Instructions:

1. Coat the inside of the slow cooker insert with the coconut oil.

2. In a medium bowl, stir together the tomato sauce and mascarpone. Coat the bottom of the insert with ½ cup of sauce.

3. Arrange several eggplant slices in a single layer, or slightly overlapping, over the sauce.

4. Top with a bit of fontina cheese, a bit of Parmesan cheese, a sprinkling of almond meal, and more sauce. Continue layering until you've used all the ingredients, ending with a layer of sauce, then cheese, and then almond meal. Cover and cook for 7 hours on low or 4 hours on high. Serve hot.

Nutrition Value:

Calories: 536

Fat: 43g

Carbs: 13g

Protein: 29g

Delicious Chili Tofu Cauliflower

Serves 4

Time: 6 hours on low

Ingredients:

- 2 tablespoons coconut oil
- 2 cups cauliflower florets
- 8 ounces firm tofu, cut into 1-inch cubes
- ½ onion, diced
- 2 cups crumbled blue cheese, divided
- 1 cup diced tomatoes, with juice
- ¼ cup all-natural spicy hot sauce (such as Frank's RedHot)
- 1 tablespoon erythritol
- 1½ teaspoons chili powder
- 1 teaspoon ground cumin
- ¼ teaspoon kosher salt
- 2 celery stalks, finely diced

Instructions:

1. In the slow cooker, combine the coconut oil, cauliflower, tofu, onion, 1 cup of blue cheese, tomatoes and their juice, hot sauce, erythritol, chili powder, cumin, and salt. Stir to mix. Cover and cook for 6 hours on low.

2. Serve the chili hot, topped with the celery and remaining 1 cup of blue cheese.

Nutrition Value:

Calories: 355

Fat: 29g

Protein: 20g

Carbs: 6g

Spinach Mayo Artichoke Dip

Serving: 20

Time: 4 hours on high

Ingredients:

- 3 garlic cloves
- ½ medium onion
- 2 cans (14 ounces) artichoke hearts
- 10 ounces chopped spinach
- 10 ounces chopped kale
- 1 cup Parmesan cheese
- 1 cup shredded mozzarella cheese
- 1 cup Greek yogurt
- ¾ sour cream
- ¼ cup mayo
- Salt
- Pepper

Instructions:

Place the artichokes, garlic and onion in a food processor and chop finely.

Transfer into a slow cooker with the rest of the ingredients.

Cook for 4 hours on high. Stir mix well, forming a paste. Serve with veggie sticks.

Nutritional Value:

Calories: 83

Fat: 9g

Carbs: 5g

Protein: 3.5g

Oregano Mascarpone Zucchini Lasagna

Serves 6
Time: 7 hours on low or 3½ hours on high
Ingredients:

- Coconut oil, for coating the slow cooker insert
- 1 pound mascarpone cheese
- 1 cup grated Parmesan cheese, divided
- 1 cup chopped spinach
- 1 large egg, beaten
- 1 teaspoon dried oregano
- ¾ teaspoon kosher salt
- ½ teaspoon freshly ground black pepper
- 1½ cups tomato sauce, divided
- 1 cup heavy (whipping) cream
- 2 medium zucchini, cut into ⅓-inch slices
- 4 cups shredded fontina cheese
- 2 tablespoons chopped fresh flat-leaf parsley

Instructions:

1. Coat the inside of the slow cooker insert with coconut oil.
2. In a medium bowl, stir together the mascarpone cheese, ½ cup of Parmesan cheese, spinach, egg, oregano, salt, and pepper.
3. In a separate bowl, stir together the tomato sauce and heavy cream. Spoon 1 cup of the sauce into the slow cooker and spread it out to coat the bottom of the insert.
4. Arrange one-third of the zucchini slices in a single layer, or slightly overlapping, over the sauce.
5. Spread one-third of the mascarpone mixture over the zucchini slices, then top with one-third of the remaining tomato sauce, followed by one-third of the fontina cheese. Repeat the layers two more times.
6. Sprinkle the remaining ½ cup of Parmesan cheese over the top. Cover and cook for 7 hours on low or 3½ hours on high. Serve hot, garnished with the parsley.

Nutrition Value:
Calories: 696
Fat: 61g
Carbs: 8g
Protein: 31g

Balsamic Artichoke Summer Dish

Serving: 4

Time: 3hours on high

Ingredients:

- 6 chopped basil leaves
- ½ cup artichoke hearts, quartered
- ¼ cup halved Kalamata olives
- ¼ cup capers
- 20 diced Roma tomatoes
- 3 tbsps. balsamic vinegar
- 3 tbsps. avocado oil
- ¾ tsp. onion powder
- ¾ tsp. sea salt
- ½ tsp. black pepper
- 2 tbsps. minced garlic

Instructions:

Combine all the ingredients in the slow cooker and mix well.

Cook for 3 hours on high, stirring the mix after every hour.

Nutritional Value

Calories: 152

Fat: 13g

Carb: 6g

Protein 8 g

Coconut Pumpkin Curry

Serves 4

Time: 6 hours on low

Ingredients:

- 2 tablespoons coconut oil, melted
- 1½ pounds extra-firm tofu, cut into 1-inch cubes
- 12 ounces cremini or button mushrooms, halved or quartered
- ½ cup diced onion
- 2 garlic cloves, minced
- 1 tablespoon grated fresh ginger
- 3 tablespoons curry powder
- 1 teaspoon ground cumin
- 1 teaspoon kosher salt
- ½ teaspoon cayenne pepper
- 1 (14-ounce) can coconut milk
- ¼ cup chopped macadamia nuts
- ¼ cup chopped fresh cilantro

Instructions:

1. Coat the inside of the slow cooker insert with the coconut oil. Add the tofu, mushrooms, onion, garlic, ginger, curry powder, cumin, salt, cayenne, and coconut milk. Cover and cook for 6 hours on low.

2. Serve hot, garnished with the macadamia nuts and cilantro.

Nutrition Value:

Calories: 350

Fat: 29g

Protein: 16g

Carbs: 11g

Balsamic-Glazed Pine Nuts Brussels Sprouts

Serves 6

Time: 6 hours on low or 3 hours on high

Ingredients:

- 1 pound Brussels sprouts, halved
- 2 tablespoons coconut oil
- Kosher salt
- Freshly ground black pepper
- 2 tablespoons unsalted butter, cubed
- 2 tablespoons balsamic vinegar
- 2 tablespoons erythritol
- 2 cups grated Parmesan cheese
- ¼ cup toasted pine nuts

Instructions:

1. In the slow cooker, combine the Brussels sprouts and coconut oil. Season with salt and pepper and stir to mix.

2. Top with the butter. Cover and cook for 6 hours on low or 3 hours on high.

3. In a small saucepan, combine the balsamic vinegar and erythritol over medium heat and bring to a boil. Reduce the heat a bit and simmer until the liquid is thick and syrupy, about 8 minutes.

4. To serve, drizzle the balsamic glaze over the Brussels sprouts and serve hot, garnished with the Parmesan cheese and pine nuts.

Nutrition Value:

Calories: 354

Fat: 28g

Carbs: 12g

Protein: 20g

Delicious Tofu & Vegetables Tofu Curry

Serves 4

Time: 6 hours on low

Ingredients:

- 2 tablespoons coconut oil
- ½ onion, diced
- 1 tablespoon minced fresh ginger
- 2 garlic cloves, minced
- 1 pound firm tofu, diced
- ½ green bell pepper, seeded and sliced
- 1 (14-ounce) can coconut milk
- ¼ cup Thai green curry paste
- 1 tablespoon erythritol
- 1 teaspoon kosher salt
- ½ teaspoon turmeric
- ¼ cup chopped fresh cilantro, for garnish

Instructions:

1. In a medium skillet, heat the coconut oil over medium-high heat.

2. Add the onion and sauté until softened, about 5 minutes.

3. Stir in the ginger and garlic and then transfer the mixture to the slow cooker.

4. Mix in the tofu, green bell pepper, coconut milk, curry paste, erythritol, salt, and turmeric. Cover and cook for 6 hours on low. Serve hot, garnished with the cilantro.

Nutrition Value

Calories: 380

Fat: 31g

Carb: 11g

Protein: 15g

KETO SLOW COOKER DESSERTS RECIPES

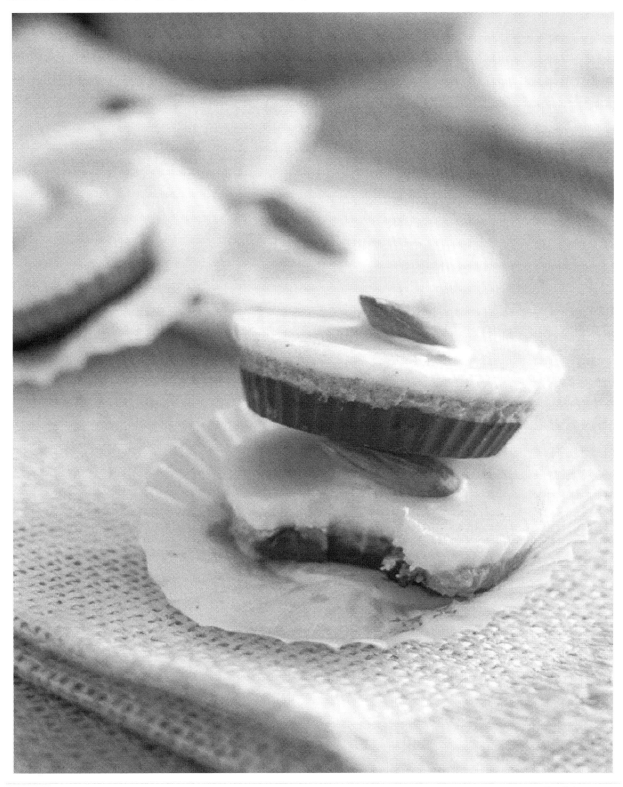

Delicious Cinnamon-Cocoa Almonds

Serves 8

Time: 2 hours on high

Ingredients:

- 3 cups raw almonds
- 3 tablespoons coconut oil, melted
- Kosher salt
- ¼ cup erythritol
- 1 tablespoon unsweetened cocoa powder
- 1 tablespoon ground cinnamon

Instructions:

1. In the slow cooker, stir together the almonds and coconut oil until the nuts are well coated. Season with salt.

2. Mix in the erythritol, cocoa powder, and cinnamon. Cover and cook for 2 hours on high, stirring every 30 minutes.

3. Transfer the nuts to a large, rimmed baking sheet and spread them out to cool quickly. Serve immediately or store in a covered container for up to 3 weeks.

Make It Paleo Simply leave out the sweetener, or replace it with a paleo-friendly sweetener, such as coconut sugar.

Nutrition Value:

Calories: 275

Fat: 23g

Carbs: 8g

Protein: 9g

Yummy Stevia Coconut Custard

Serves 8

Time: 5 hours on low, plus 1 to 2 hours to cool

Ingredients:

- 1 tablespoon coconut oil
- 8 large eggs, lightly beaten
- 4 cups canned coconut milk
- 1 cup erythritol or 1 teaspoon stevia powder
- 2 teaspoons stevia powder
- 1 teaspoon coconut extract

Instructions:

1. Generously coat the inside of the slow cooker insert with the coconut oil.

2. In the insert, stir together the eggs, coconut milk, erythritol, stevia powder, and coconut extract until well combined.

3. Cover and cook for 5 hours on low. Turn off the cooker and let cool in the slow cooker for 1 to 2 hours.

4. Serve immediately or refrigerate for up to 3 days and serve chilled.

Nutrition Value:

Calories: 375

Fat: 35g

Carbs: 7g

Protein: 9g

Delicious Almond Coconut Brownie

Time: 4 hours 10 minutes

Serving: 10

Ingredients:

- 2 eggs
- 1/3 cup water
- 2 tsp vanilla extract
- 1/2 cup coconut oil, melted
- 1/2 cup coconut milk, unsweetened
- 2 tsp baking soda
- 2 tsp baking powder
- 3/4 cup cocoa powder, unsweetened
- 1 cup coconut sugar
- 2 cups almond flour
- 1 tsp salt

Instructions:

Grease slow cooker with coconut oil.

Combine together all ingredients and add in the slow cooker.

Cover slow cooker with lid and cook on low for 4 minutes.

Allow cooling mixture for half hour.

Scoop out mixture with large spoon and form into balls.

Serve and enjoy.

Nutritional Value :

Calories 289

Fat 26 g

Carb: 11.5 g

Protein 7.5 g

Vanilla Cocoa Pudding

Time: 3 hours 20 minutes

Serving : 6

Ingredients:

- 5 eggs
- 1/3 cup almond flour
- 2/3 cup stevia
- 4 tbsp cocoa powder, unsweetened
- 1 tsp vanilla extract
- 2 tbsp instant coffee
- 1/2 cup heavy cream
- 2 oz unsweetened chocolate, chopped
- 3/4 cup butter, cut into pieces
- 1/8 Tsp salt

Instructions:

Spray slow cooker form inside using cooking spray.

In a small saucepan, melt chocolate and butter over low heat and set aside to cool.

In a small bowl, whisk together vanilla, coffee, and heavy cream. In a small bowl, combine almond flour, cocoa, and salt.

Add eggs into the large bowl and beat until creamy then slowly add sweetener and beat again until thickened.

Now slowly add chocolate and butter mixture and stir well. Stir in almond flour, cocoa, and salt mixture. Slowly add vanilla, coffee and cream mixture and beat over low speed to well combine.

Pour batter into the slow cooker. Cook on low for 3 hours. Cut cake into the pieces and serve.

Nutritional Value

Calories: 413

Fat: 39 g

Carb: 3.7 g

Protein 9 g

Gluten Free Coconut Lemon Cake

Time: 3 hours 10 minutes

Serving : 8

Ingredients:

- 2 eggs
- 1 1/2 cups almond flour
- 2 lemon zest
- 2 tbsp lemon juice
- 1/2 cup whipping cream
- 1/2 cup butter, melted
- 2 tsp baking powder
- 6 tbsp Swerve
- 1/2 cup coconut flour

Instructions:

In a medium bowl, combine together almond flour, baking powder, swerve, and coconut flour.

In a large bowl, whisk together eggs, lemon zest, lemon juice, whipping cream, and butter.

Add dry mixture into the wet and fold until well combined.

Pour batter into the slow cooker and cook on high for 3 hours.

Cut into pieces and serve warm.

Nutritional Value

Calories 350

Fat 32 g

Carb: 11 g

Protein 7.6 g

Rich Flavor Grain-Free Brownies

Serve: 12 brownies

Time: Cook: 4 hours on low

Ingredients:

- ¼ cup unsalted butter, plus more for coating the slow cooker insert
- 4 ounces unsweetened chocolate, chopped
- 1½ cups almond flour
- ½ cup unsweetened cocoa powder
- ¼ cup coconut flour
- 2 teaspoons baking powder
- ¼ teaspoon fine sea salt
- 1 large ripe avocado, peeled, pitted, and mashed
- ¼ cup heavy (whipping) cream
- 3 large eggs, lightly beaten
- ¾ cup erythritol
- ¾ teaspoon stevia powder
- ¾ cup coarsely chopped walnuts

Instructions:

1. Coat the bottom and sides of the slow cooker insert with butter, then line the bottom with parchment or wax paper (trace the bottom of the insert on the parchment and then cut it out).

2. In a small, microwave-safe bowl, combine ¼ cup of butter and the chocolate. Heat for 30-second intervals on high, stirring after each interval, until the chocolate is melted and the ingredients are fully incorporated.

3. In a medium bowl, stir together the almond flour, cocoa powder, coconut flour, baking powder, and salt. In a large bowl, mix the avocado and heavy cream until smooth.

5. Add the eggs, erythritol, and stevia and mix to combine. Mix in the melted chocolate until incorporated.

6. Add the dry ingredients to the wet ingredients and mix until incorporated. Stir in the walnuts.

7. Transfer the mixture to the slow cooker and spread evenly. Cover and cook for 4 hours on low. Let cool for about 30 minutes in the slow cooker. Run a knife around the edge and then lift out of the insert. Cut into pieces and serve at room temperature.

Nutrition Value: Calories: 229; Fat: 21g; Carbs: 8g; Protein: 10g

Coconut Toasted Almond Cheesecake

Serves 8

Time: Cook: 4 hours on low or 2 hours on high, & time to chill

Ingredients:

- FOR THE CRUST
- 1 cup toasted almonds, ground to a meal
- 1 large egg, lightly beaten
- 2 tablespoons coconut oil, melted
- 1 teaspoon stevia powder
- 1 cup water
- FOR THE FILLING
- 2 large eggs
- 2 (8-ounce) packages cream cheese, at room temperature
- ¾ cup almond butter
- ¼ cup coconut cream
- 1 teaspoon pure almond extract
- ¾ cup erythritol
- 1 tablespoon coconut flour
- 2 teaspoons stevia powder

Instructions:

TO MAKE THE CRUST

1. In a medium bowl, mix the almond meal, egg, coconut oil, and stevia powder. Press the mixture into the bottom of a baking pan that fits into your slow cooker (make sure there is room to lift the pan out). Many pans could work, depending on the size and shape of your slow cooker. Pour the water into the slow cooker insert. Place the pan in the cooker.

TO MAKE THE FILLING

1. In a large bowl, beat the eggs, then beat in the cream cheese, almond butter, coconut cream, almond extract, erythritol, coconut flour, and stevia powder. Pour the mixture over the crust. Cover and cook for 4 hours on low or 2 hours on high.

2. When finished, turn off the slow cooker and let the cheesecake sit inside until cooled to room temperature, up to 3 hours.

3. Remove the pan from the slow cooker and refrigerate until chilled, about 2 hours more. Serve chilled.

Nutrition Value: Calories: 538; Fat: 51g; Carbs: 12g; Protein: 14g

Shredded Coconut-Raspberry Cake

Serves 10

Time: Cook: 3 hours, plus 3 to 4 hours to cool

Ingredients:

- ½ cup melted coconut oil, plus more for coating the slow cooker insert
- 2 cups almond flour
- 1 cup unsweetened shredded coconut
- 1 cup erythritol or 1 teaspoon stevia powder
- ¼ cup unsweetened, unflavored protein powder
- 2 teaspoons baking soda
- ¼ teaspoon fine sea salt
- 4 large eggs, lightly beaten
- ¾ cup canned coconut milk
- 1 teaspoon coconut extract
- 1 cup raspberries, fresh or frozen

Instructions:

1. Generously coat the inside of the slow cooker insert with coconut oil.

2. In a large bowl, stir together the almond flour, coconut, erythritol, protein powder, baking soda, and sea salt.

3. Whisk in the eggs, coconut milk, ½ cup of coconut oil, and coconut extract.

4. Gently fold in the raspberries.

5. Transfer the batter to the prepared slow cooker, cover, and cook for 3 hours on low. Turn off the slow cooker and let the cake cool for several hours, to room temperature. Serve at room temperature.

Nutrition Value:

Calories: 405

Fat: 38g

Carbs: 8g

Protein: 11g

Vanilla Chocolate Walnut Fudge

Serves 12

Time : 2 hours on low, plus 3 hours to cool, overnight to chill

Ingredients:

- Coconut oil, for coating the slow cooker insert and a baking dish
- 1 cup canned coconut milk
- 4 ounces unsweetened chocolate, chopped
- 1 cup erythritol
- 2 teaspoons stevia powder
- ¼ teaspoon fine sea salt
- 2 teaspoons pure vanilla extract
- 1 cup chopped toasted walnuts

Instructions:

1. Generously coat the inside of the slow cooker insert with coconut oil.

2. In a large bowl, whisk the coconut milk into a uniform consistency. Add the chocolate, erythritol, stevia powder, and sea salt. Stir to mix well. Pour into the slow cooker. Cover and cook for 2 hours on low.

3. When finished, stir in the vanilla.

4. Let the fudge sit in the slow cooker, with the lid off, until it cools to room temperature, about 3 hours.

5. Coat a large baking dish with coconut oil and set aside.

6. Stir the fudge until it becomes glossy, about 10 minutes.

7. Stir in the walnuts. Transfer the mixture to the prepared baking dish and smooth it into an even layer with a rubber spatula. Refrigerate overnight. Serve chilled, cut into small pieces.

Nutrition Value:

Calories: 128

Fat: 13g

Carbs: 4g

Protein: 3g

Delicious Chocolate Peanut Butter Fudge

Serves 12

Time: 2 hours on low, plus 4 hours to chill

Ingredients:

- Coconut oil, for coating the slow cooker insert
- 1½ cups heavy (whipping) cream
- 1 cup all-natural peanut butter
- 1 tablespoon unsalted butter, melted
- 1 teaspoon pure vanilla extract
- 4 ounces unsweetened chocolate, chopped
- ½ cup erythritol
- 1 teaspoon stevia powder

Instructions:

1. Generously coat the inside of the slow cooker insert with coconut oil.

2. In the slow cooker, stir together the heavy cream, peanut butter, butter, vanilla, chocolate, erythritol, and stevia. Cover and cook for 2 hours on low, stirring occasionally.

3. Line a small, rimmed baking sheet with parchment or wax paper.

4. Transfer the cooked fudge to the prepared sheet and refrigerate for at least 4 hours.

5. Cut into squares and serve chilled.

Nutrition Value:

Calories: 246

Fat: 23g

Carbs: 7g

Protein: 9g

Creamy Low-Carb Vanilla Cheesecake

Serves 8

Time: 4 hours on low or 2 hours on high, plus time to chill

Ingredients:

- FOR THE CRUST
- 1 cup toasted walnuts, ground to a meal
- 1 large egg, lightly beaten
- 2 tablespoons coconut oil, melted
- 1 teaspoon stevia powder
- 1 cup water
- FOR THE FILLING
- 2 large eggs
- 2 (8-ounce) packages cream cheese, at room temperature
- ¼ cup heavy (whipping) cream
- 2 teaspoons pure vanilla extract
- ½ cup erythritol
- 1 tablespoon coconut flour
- ½ teaspoon stevia powder

Instructions:

TO MAKE THE CRUST

1. In a medium bowl, mix the walnut meal, egg, coconut oil, and stevia powder. Press the mixture into the bottom of a baking pan that fits into your slow cooker (make sure there is room to lift the pan out). An oval baking dish, round cake pan, or loaf pan could all work, depending on the size and shape of your slow cooker.

2. Pour the water into the slow cooker insert. Place the pan in the cooker.

TO MAKE THE FILLING

1. In a large bowl, beat the eggs, then beat in the cream cheese, heavy cream, vanilla, erythritol, coconut flour, and stevia powder. Pour the mixture over the crust. Cover and cook for 4 hours on low or 2 hours on high.

2. When finished, turn off the cooker and let the cheesecake sit inside until cooled to room temperature, up to 3 hours. Remove the pan from the slow cooker and refrigerate until chilled, about 2 hours more. Serve chilled.

Nutrition Value: Calories: 338; Fat: 33g; Carbs: 5g; Protein: 7g

CONCLUSION

Thank you once again for purchasing my book, I hope you have enjoyed cooking with this book .

If you don't mind, I would like to ask if you could please kindly leave me an honest review on amazon .

Thank you and good luck!

Emma Green

Made in the USA
Middletown, DE
02 July 2019